PATHOPHYSIOLOGY AND COMPLICATIONS OF DIABETES MELLITUS

Edited by **Oluwafemi O. Oguntibeju**

Pathophysiology and Complications of Diabetes Mellitus

http://dx.doi.org/10.5772/3460
Edited by Oluwafemi O. Oguntibeju

Contributors

Shahriar Ahmadpour, Manjunatha B. K. Goud, Sarsina O. Devi, Bhavna Nayal, Saidunnisa Begum, Daniela Pedicino, Ada Francesca Giglio, Vincenzo Alessandro Galiffa, Francesco Trotta, Giovanna Liuzzo, Božidar Vujičić, Tamara Turk, Željka Crnčević-Orlić, Gordana Đorđević, Sanjin Rački, G. Malathi, V. Shanthi, Michal Straka, Michaela Straka-Trapezanlidis

Published by InTech

Janeza Trdine 9, 51000 Rijeka, Croatia

Publishing Process Manager Oliver Kurelic
Typesetting InTech DTP Team
Cover InTech Design Team

Additional hard copies can be obtained from orders@intechopen.com

Pathophysiology and Complications of Diabetes Mellitus,
Edited by Oluwafemi O. Oguntibeju
p. cm.
ISBN 978-953-51-0833-7

For EU product safety concerns:
IN TECH d.o.o., Prolaz Marije Krucifikse Kozulić 3, 51000 Rijeka, Croatia, info@intechopen.com or visit our website at intechopen.com.

Meet the editor

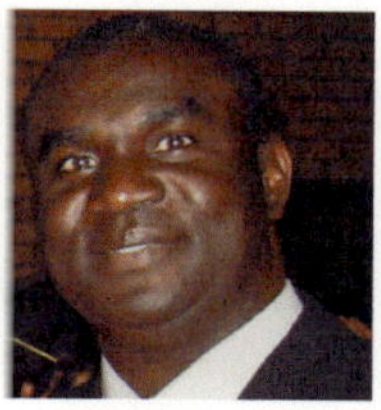

Prof Oluwafemi O. Oguntibeju is an Associate Professor and Group Leader (Nutrition and Chronic Disease Research Unit) at the Oxidative Stress Research Centre in the Department of Biomedical Sciences, Faculty of Health & Wellness, Cape Peninsula University of Technology Bellville, South Africa. He lectures and supervises postgraduate students and collaborates with national and international scientists. Over the years, he has been involved in the field of nutrition and HIV/AIDS and related-public health issues but more recently on diabetes. He has published over 90 scientific papers in peer-reviewed journals, presented over 30 papers at national and international conferences and reviewed manuscripts for over 30 international scientific journals. He has received various awards such as the Gold Research Excellence Award at his current university. Prof O. O. Oguntibeju is a National Research Foundation (NRF) C-rated researcher and holds a master degree in Biochemistry from the University of Ibadan, Nigeria and a doctoral degree in Biomedical Science at the Central University of Technology, Bloemfontein, South Africa. He is a Chartered Scientist (CSci, UK) and Fellow of the Institute of Biomedical Science, London. He enjoys reading and music and he is married to Faustina and has four children.

Contents

Preface

The book "Pathophysiology and complications of diabetes mellitus" is organized into six chapters and focused mainly on the pathophysiology and complications of diabetes mellitus. This book provides expert contributions in terms of experience and scientific knowledge on the subject. Students, scientists, teaching academics and various health professionals would find this book very informative and useful. The references cited in each chapter definitely act as additional and vital source of information for readers.

Oluwafemi O. Oguntibeju
Department of Biomedical Sciences, Faculty of Health & Wellness Sciences,
Cape Peninsula University of Technology, Bellville,
South Africa

Chapter 1

CNS Complications of Diabetes Mellitus Type 1 (Type 1 Diabetic Encephalopathy)

Shahriar Ahmadpour

Additional information is available at the end of the chapter

http://dx.doi.org/10.5772/49990

1. Introduction

Diabetes mellitus type1 (T1D) or insulin dependent diabetes mellitus (IDDM) is an endocrine metabolic disorder which is defined by absolute or partial lack of insulin and hyperglycemia (1).Traditionally the complications of diabetes were classified as acute complications like diabetic keto acidosis (DKA) and chronic complications. Chronic complications comprise vascular and nonvascular complications. The vascular complications are further subdivided into microvascular (retinopathy, neuropathy, and nephropathy) and macrovascular complications (coronary artery disease, CAD, and cerebrovascular disease) (2). Despite the first record of diabetes-related cognitive dysfunctions in 1922 (3), for a long period diabetic nephropathy, peripheral neuropathy, and retinopathy were considered as late diabetes microvascular complications and it was believed that central nervous system (CNS) as an insulin independent organ, spares from diabetic complications. However in recent decades studies have provided evidence that indicate the deleterious effects of T1DM on structure and functions of the brain (4-6). Duration related or chronic effects of T1DM on the brain, T1DM encephalopathy, are manifested at the all levels of CNS from microscopic to macroscopic level. Macroscopically neuroimaging studies have demonstrated a high incidence of abnormalities like temporal lobe sclerosis, decreases in white matter volume in parahippocampus, temporal and frontal lobes as well as decreased gray matter volumes of the thalami, hippocampi, and insular cortex, decreased gray matter densities of superior and middle temporal gyri and frontal gyri (7, 8).In experimental models of T1DM a vast spectrum of neuronal changes have been reported. These pathological abnormalities include synaptic and neuronal alterations, degeneration, increased cerebral microvasular permeability, and neuronal loss which collectively can lead to cognitive impairment and higher risk of development dementia (9-11). Although the mechanisms through which hyperglycemia might mediate these effects are not completely understood it seems hyperglycemia increases oxidative stress in mitochondria and subsequent free radicals generation. Increased free radicals damage cellular membrane (lipid per oxidation) and initiate death signaling pathways (12-14). One of the most sensitive regions of the brain to the metabolic disorders and oxidative stress is hippocampus (15). The hippocampus itself is divided into two interlocking sectors, the dentate gyrus and the hippocampus proper (cornu ammonis). The dentate gyrus has three layers: (1) the granular layer containing the densely packed cell bodies of the granule cells; (2) the molecular layer formed by the intertwining apical dendrites of the granule cells and their afferents; (3) the polymorph layer in the hilus of the dentate gyrus containing the initial segments of the granule-cell axons as they gather to form the glutamergic mossy fiber bundle. Hippocampus proper as an archeocortiacl structure has been divided into seven layers as follows: (1) The alveus; containing the axons of the pyramidal cells (2) the stratum oriens, a layer between the alveus and the pyramidal cell bodies which contains the basal dendrites of the pyramidal cells (3) the stratum pyramidal (4) the stratum radiatum and (5) the stratum lacunosum/molecular which are, respectively, the proximal and distal segments of the apical dendritic tree. In the CA3 field an additional layer is recognized: the stratum lucidum, interposed between the pyramidal cell bodies and the stratum radiatum, receiving the mossy-fibers input from the dentate granule cells. Each CA3 giant pyramidal neuron with large dendretic spines receive as many as10-50 mossy fibers from dentate gyrus, and send their axons into the fimbria. New memory formation and consolidation process of events by hippocampus depend on the integrity of hippocampus internal circuits (16, 17) (fig1).

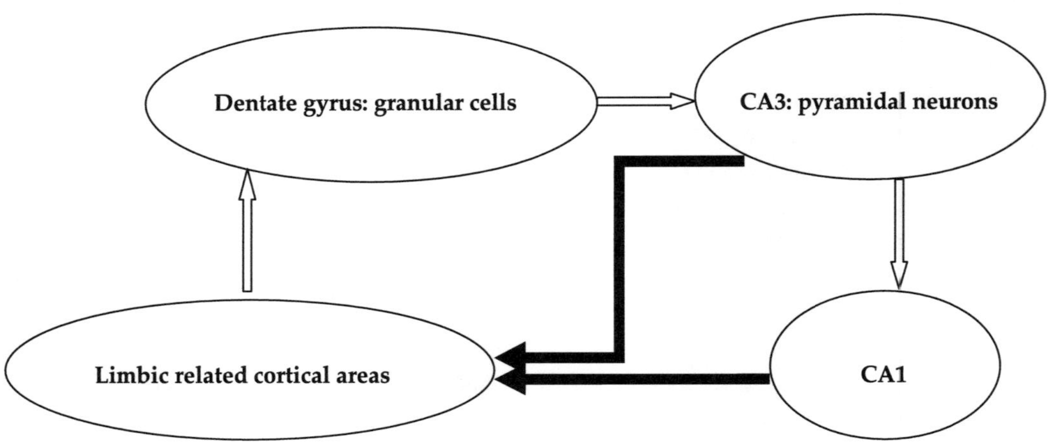

Figure 1. Functional circuits of hippocampus. Inputs from extensive cortical and subcortical areas reach dentate gyrus. Mossy fibers, axons of granular cells, synapse with CA3 pyramidal neurons.CA3 pyramidal neurons send collateral to CA1.Axons from these two regions reach limbic related regions.

Hippocampus structural complexity has made it vulnerable to the many pathological conditions such as diabetes mellitus type1 (18). It is a crucial part of the limbic system, which plays a pivotal role in memory formation, emotional, adaptive and reproductive behaviors (16 17 and19). Studies have shown that cell proliferation continues in granular layer of DG constantly. This unique neuronal renew is necessary for memory formation (20, 21). Any factor disturbing the balance between neuronal proliferations /death may result to memory and learning impairment (22). Studies have demonstrated that experimental diabetes causes decreased granular cells proliferation and neuronal death (necrosis / apoptosis) in CA3 and DG regions (23).Although neuronal death has been considered as the main leading cause of diabetic CNS and peripheral neuropathies the mode of neuronal death in T1DM has remained as a matter of controversy (24, 25, and 26). Neuronal death has been known as a common feature of neurodegenerative diseases like Alzheimer and diabetes (27).Studies have suggested free radicals and glutamate excitotoxicity as the main driving causes of neuronal death in diabetic paradigm (27-28). Interestingly these factors have been implicated in another mysterious and different type of neuronal death which is called "Dark" neuron. This kind of neuron has been reported in various pathological conditions likes stroke, epilepsy, hypoglycemia, aging and spreading depression phenomena (SD) .On the other hand, dark neuron formation has been reported in stress full conditions such as acute physical stress, normal ageing process in cerebellum and postmortem (nonenzymatic). All of these pathologic conditions cause disturbance in ion gradient (Na/K ATP_{ase} pump), and increases excitatory neurotransmitters like glutamate (27, 28).Despite the role of hyperglycemia in increasing oxidative stress and extracellular level of glutamate in hippocampus, there is little information about the effect(s) of a chronic endogenous stressor like diabetes type 1 on dark neuron formation in DG granule cells. In spite of new therapies like intranasal insulin, C peptide and antioxidants (9) diabetic central neuropathy and its underlying mechanisms have remained far from fully understood.

Purpose: Obviously understanding the neuronal death mechanisms as a common feature of neurodegenerative diseases like Alzheimer and diabetes would contribute to better understanding of its pathophysiology and new treatment approaches. As stated before dark neurons can form in enzyme-independent condition. Therefore, there may be a need to revise the cell death concept and types. This study was conducted to clarify the following questions:(1) Does hyperglycemia lead to dark neurons formation in granule layer of DG?(2) What is the nature and entity of the ultrastructural changes?

2. Materials and method

Experimental diabetes mellitus induction

Streptozotocin is a glucosamine–nitrosourea compound isolated from Streptomyces achromogenes. As an alkylating agent it interferes with glucose transport. It is taken up into beta cells of pancreas via the specific transporter, GLU-2, inducing multiple DNA strands breaks. Because of the absence of The GLUT-2 glucose, STZ direct effects on the brain tissue is eliminated following systemic administration (29).

Induction of experimental diabetes

This study was carried out on male Wistar rats (age eight weeks, body weight 240–260 g, n=6 per group).All rats maintained in animal house and allowed free access to drinking water and standard rodent diet. Experiments performed during the light period of cycle and conducted in accordance with Regional Committee of Ethic complied with the regulations of the European Convention on Vertebrate Animals Protection (2005).We considered fasting blood glucose (FBG) >250 mg/dL as a diabetic. T1D was induced by a single intraperitoneal (IP) injection of STZ (Sigma Chemical,St. Louis, Mo) at a dose of 60 mg/kg dissolved in saline (control animals were injected with saline only) (30).Four days after the STZ injection, FBG was determined in blood samples of tail veins by a digital glucometer (BIONIME, Swiss). In the end of eight weeks, the animals were anesthetized by chloroform. Then perfusion was done transcardially with 100 mL of saline followed by 200 mL of fixative containing 2% glutaraldehyde and 2% paraformaldehyde in 0.1 M phosphate buffer (pH 7.4). The harvested brains were post-fixed in the same fixative for two weeks. Then the brain further processed through graded ethanol followed by xylene and paraffin. Serial coronal sections (thickness 10 μm) were made through the entire extent of hippocampus in left and right hemispheres using a microtome.

Transmission electron microscopy (TEM)

The hippocampi (two for each group) were removed and processed as follows briefly: washing in phosphate buffer 0.1 M (pH 7.4), fixation in 1% osmium tetroxide,dehydration by graded acetones (50, 70, 80, 90 each 20 minutes, and 100 three changes ×30 minutes), infiltration by resin/acetone (1/3 overnight, 1/1 8 hours and 3/1 8 hours), resin (overnight) and embedding, thick sectioning, thin sectioning (60–90 nm), staining with uranyl acetate and lead citrate. To identify DG region, the semi thin were stained by 1% Toluidine Blue. Finally, electron micrographs were taken by EM900 (Zeiss, Germany) equipped to TFPO camera.

Gallyas' method (dark neurons staining)

Gallyas' method is a useful method for detecting of DNs. This argyrophil staining is based on the damage in cytoskeleton and DNs show characteristic morphological features like shrunken dark somata and dendrites (28).Four sections from each animal (16 sections per group) were selected by uniform random sampling. Dark neurons staining was done as our previous study (27) and follows as briefly: (a) random systematically selection of paraffin embedded sections, (b) dehydration in a graded 1-propanol series, (c) incubation at 560C for 16 hours in an esterifying solution consisting of 1.2% sulphuric acid, (d) 1-propanol(98%), (e) treatments in 8% acetic acid (10 minutes), (f) developing in a silicotungstate physical developer, (g) development termination by washing in 1% acetic acid (30 minutes), and (h) dehydration. The superior and inferior blades of the dentate gyrus were studied and pictures were taken by Olympus microscope (BX51, Japan) equipped with Motic Image plus 2 software (Motic China Group, LTD). Counting of DNs was carried out according to the stereological bases and therefore only cell bodies were counted (26).

Statistical analysis

All data are expressed as mean±SD. Statistical comparison for the number of DNs between two groups was made using Student t-test. Statistically significant difference was accepted at the $p<0.05$ level.

3. Results

The day 4 after STZ injection, rats were severely diabetic as indicated by their elevated plasma glucose (567.92±45.20 mg/dL) while plasma glucose of control group showed normoglycemic range (101±6.310 mg/dL) ($p<0.001$) (fig2). Diabetic rats also exhibited obvious signs of diabetes namely: polyuria and polydipsia.

Counting the DNs

The numbers of DNs in diabetic animals were counted 223±25 and those of normal group counted5.75±4.34. The comparison between the numbers of DNs in two groups showed significant level of difference ($p<0.05$) (Figure 2

Light microscopy findings

Dark neurons (DNs) in DG granular layer of STZ-induced diabetic group showed preserved cell integrity , detached from surrounding tissues, high darkly brown stained somata and degenerated axons (Figure 3-6).Filamentous (thread like) structures were noticed in soma and neuritis (Figure 4). Some granular cells showed small mitochondrion size brown grain in their perikarya (Figure 5). In control animals, some scattered DNs were also found in DG granular layer, while surrounding normal neurons were not stained (Figure 7).Staining by toluidine blue showed some neurons were deeply stained (hyperbasophilia) (figure8,9).

TEM findings

Characterization of neuronal death was according to our previous study, hence chromatin changes like clumping, margination and condensation was considered the most important evidence of non-necrotic death. Of course, other morphological characters such as cell shrinkage and dark appearance were considered. Integrity of neuronal membrane preserved in most of cases (Figs 10–14).Chromatin clumping, condensation and margination were noticed in diabetic group. The pattern of chromatin changes showed some differences. Tiny and dispersed chromatin clump in electron dense nucleus and nucleolus without chromatin adherence were seen in some dark appearance neuron(figs10,12,13) while in some chromatin clumping was more conspicuous and nucleus appearance was lighter (fig14).Other morphological changes included: reduced inter-organelles spaces, electron dense appearance, shrinkage, detachment from surrounding tissues, degenerating axon(figs11,12) and apoptotic-body (14).Swelled mitochondria were observed in cytoplasm of shrunken dark neurons (fig10). In control animals some healthy looking neurons with increased electrondensity and apoptotic bodies were observed (14). The normal healthy neuron showed normal dispersed and light chromatin (fig 14).

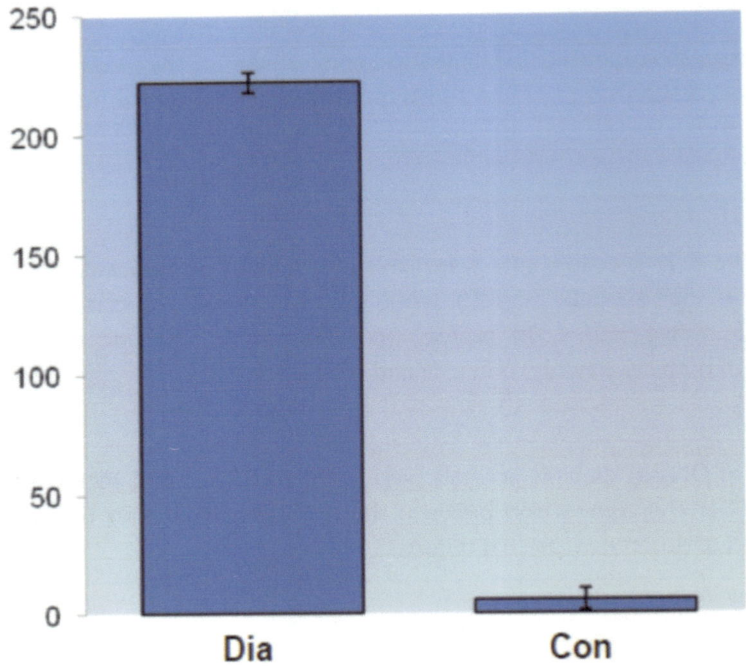

Figure 2. Counting of DNs in diabetic animals (Dia) showed significant level of difference to control group (Con). *$p<0.05$.

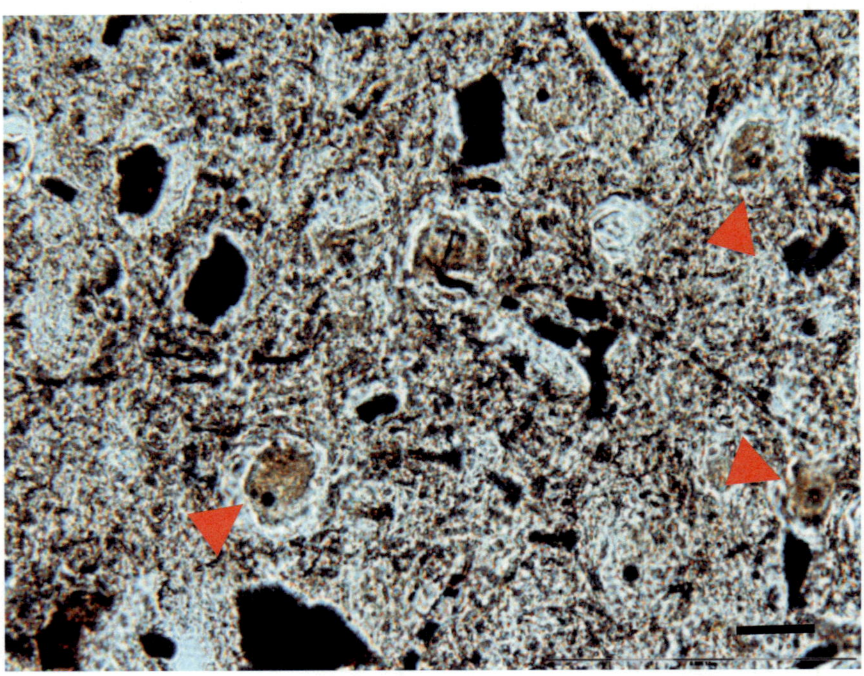

Figure 3. Reversible type of dark neurons are scattered between some dark neuron. These neurons are characterized with light brown color that is indicative of recovering phase (arrowheads). Scale bar 5 μm

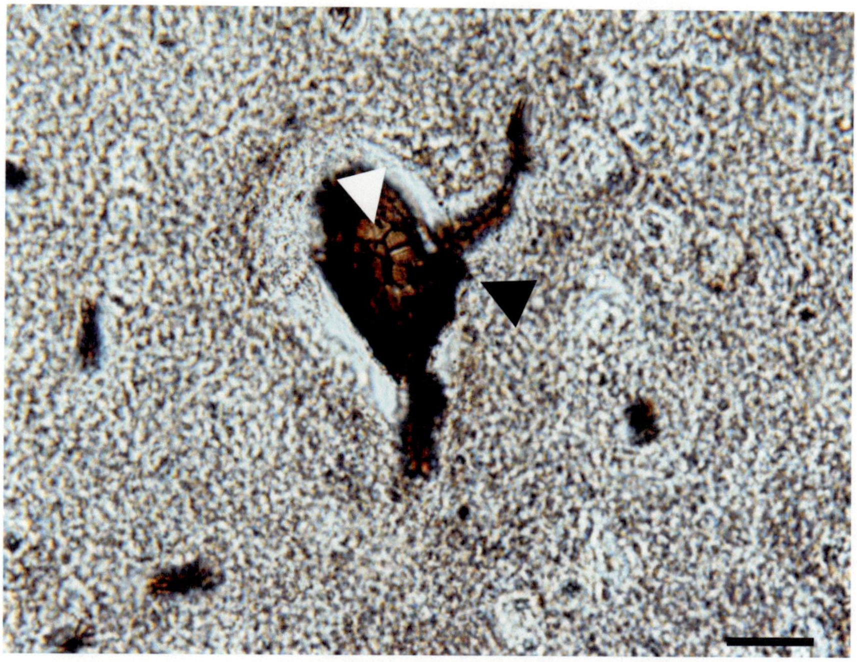

Figure 4. Fig4: A DN in the granular layer of diabetic group stained darkly brown (center). Soma of this DN shows some thread like structures (white arrow). An axosomatic synapse is also seen (right arrow). Scale bar 5 μm.

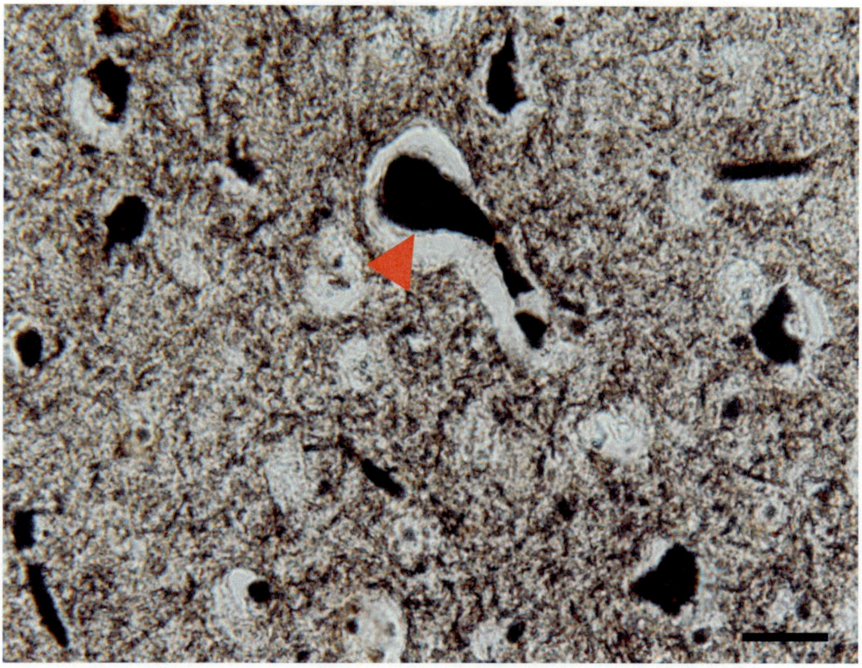

Figure 5. Dark neuron. Highly dark stained degenerated neurons. In center a dark neuron (red arrowhead) and numerous degenerated neuronal particles are seen. Diabetic group. Scale bar 5 μm

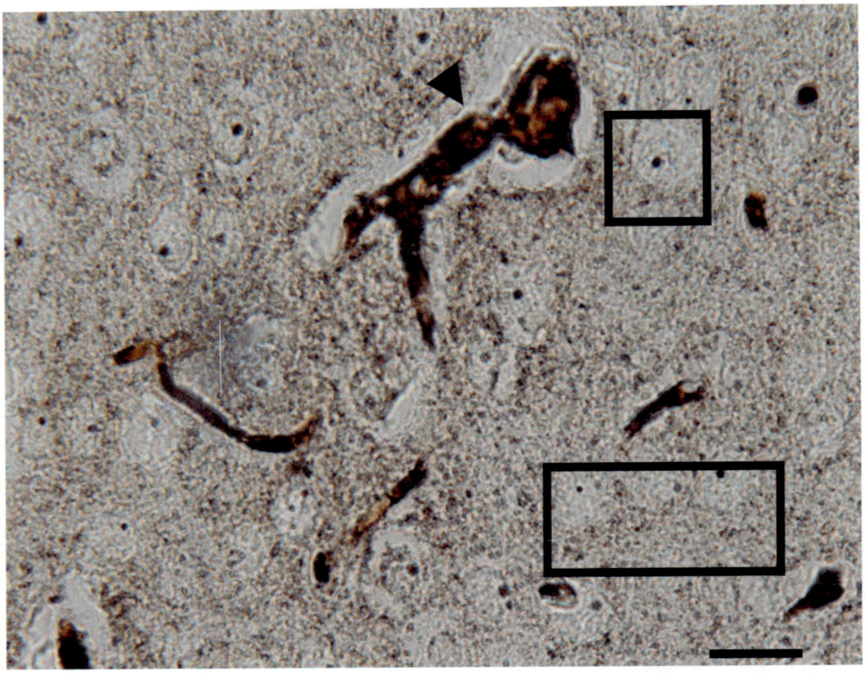

Figure 6. A DN stained by Gallyas' method. Somata and axon stained intensely (arrowhead). DN is detached from surrounding tissues and scattered among healthy neuron (windows). Scale bar 5 μm.

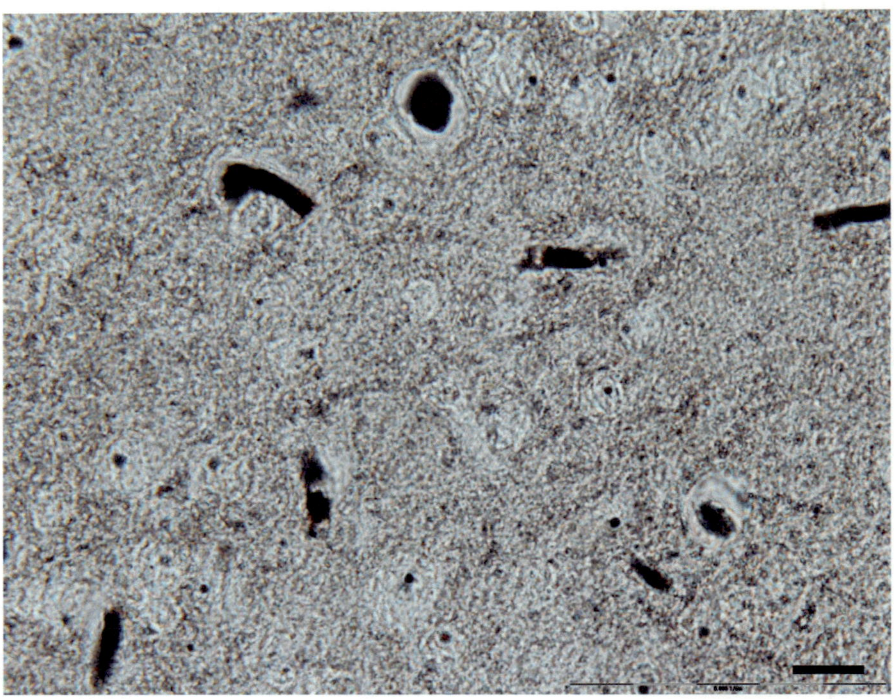

Figure 7. DG granule cells in control group. DNs (arrow) dispersed in the granular layer. Scale bar25μm

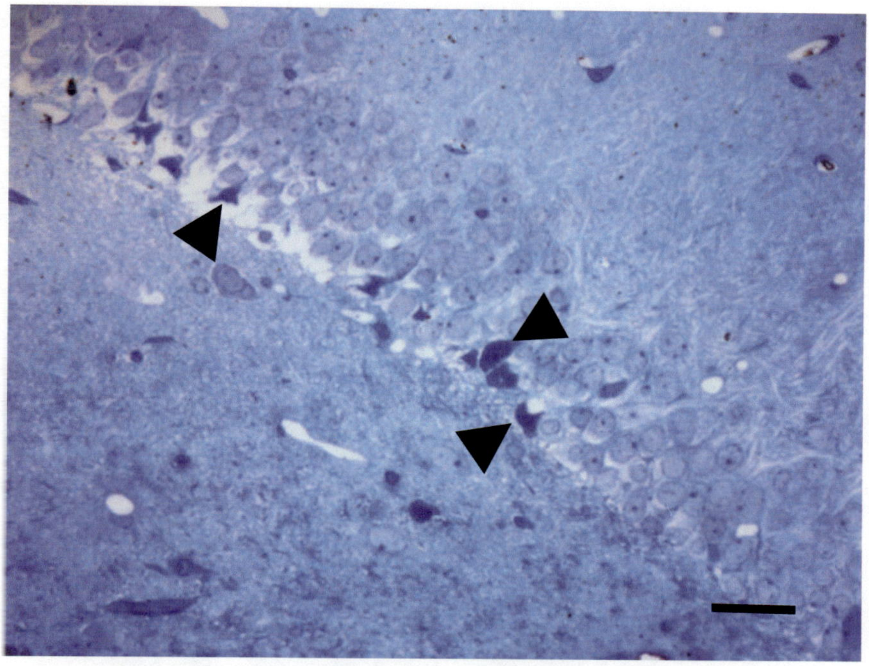

Figure 8. Semi thin sections (1μm) stained by toluidine blue. Arrows indicate dark neuron among the healthy granular layer cells of DG (control). Scale bar 25μm

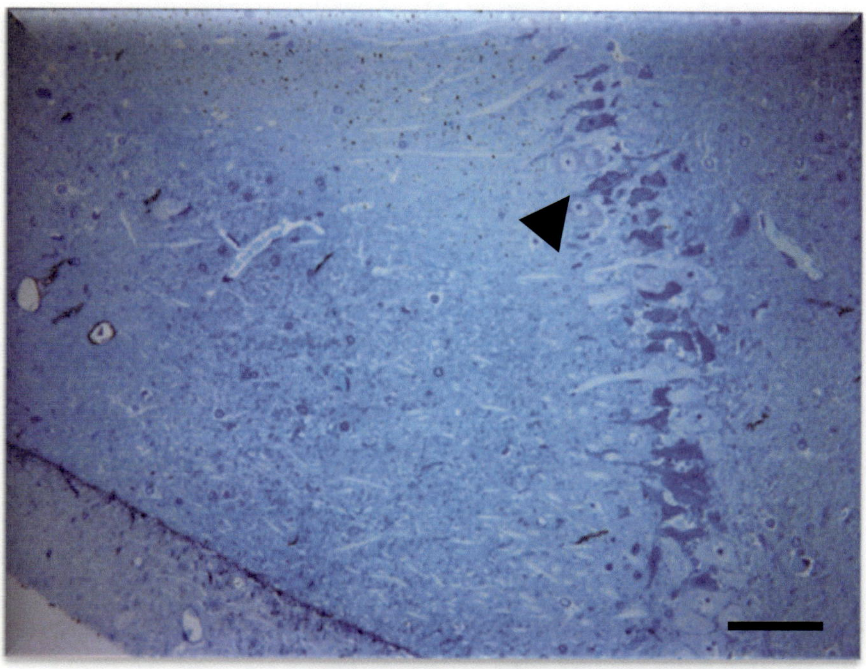

Figure 9. Semi thin sections (1μm) stained by toluidine blue. Arrow indicates normal neuron among the dark, hyperbasophilic neurons of DG. Scale bar 25μm

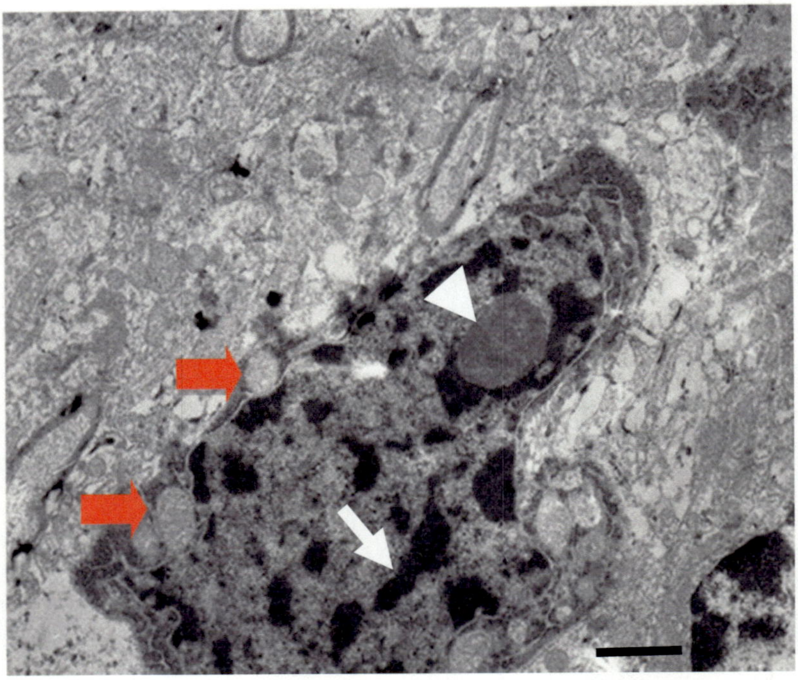

Figure 10. A DN in diabetic rats. Chromatin condensation,margination and clumping (white arrow), swollen mitochondria (arrows, right and left) are seen around the nucleus. Scale bar 2 μm.

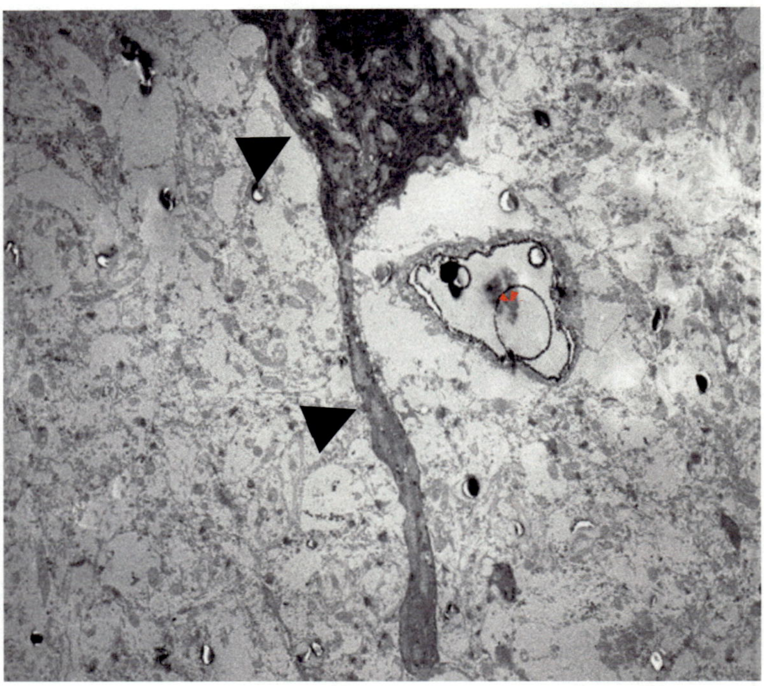

Figure 11. A DN in diabetic rats with degeneratedaxon (long arrow), dark perikarya (short arrow). Degenerative vacuolization has occurred around the DN and a vessel (star). Scale bar 5 μm.

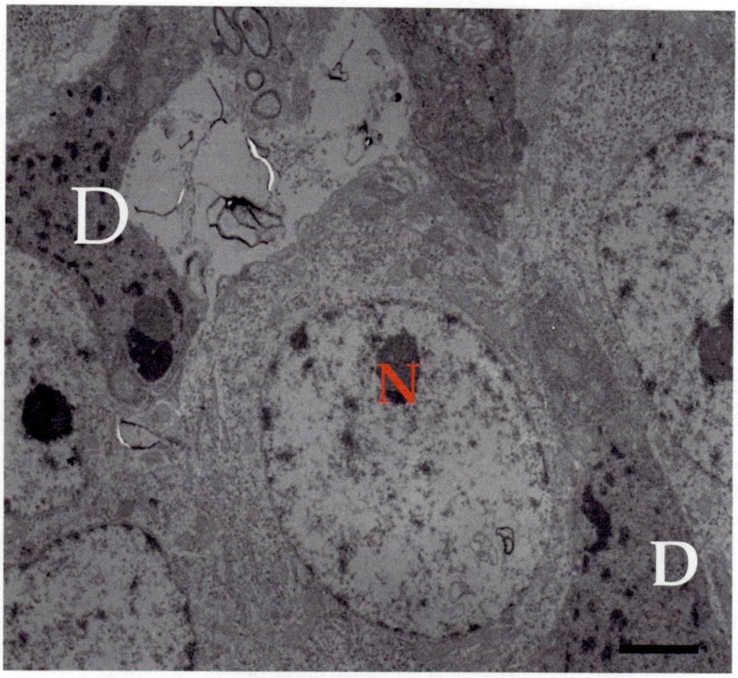

Figure 12. Normal neuron (center) and its nucleolus (N).Two dark neurons (D) with chromatin clumping. A large mass of chromatin is attached to nucleolus. Scale bar2μm

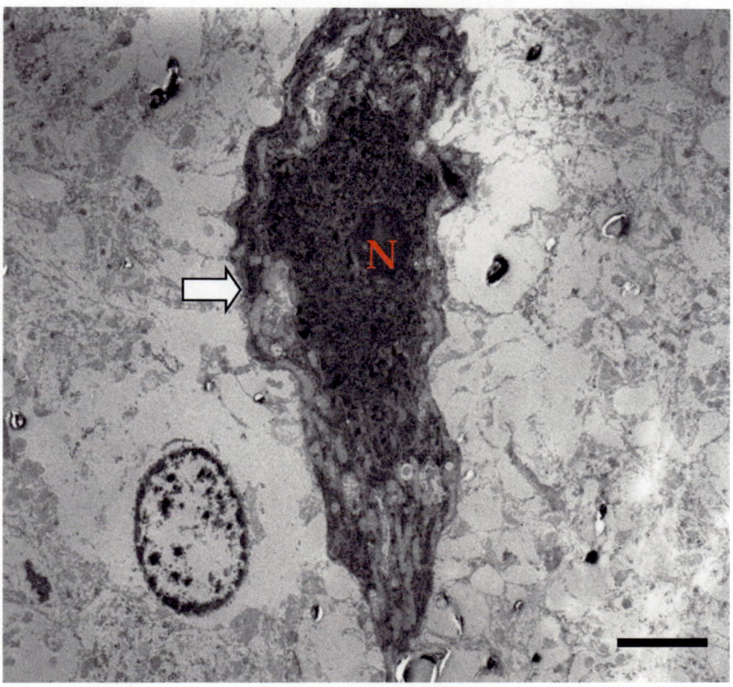

Figure 13. A dark neuron (white arrow).The pattern of chromatin clumping and nucleolus is different. Scale bar 4μm

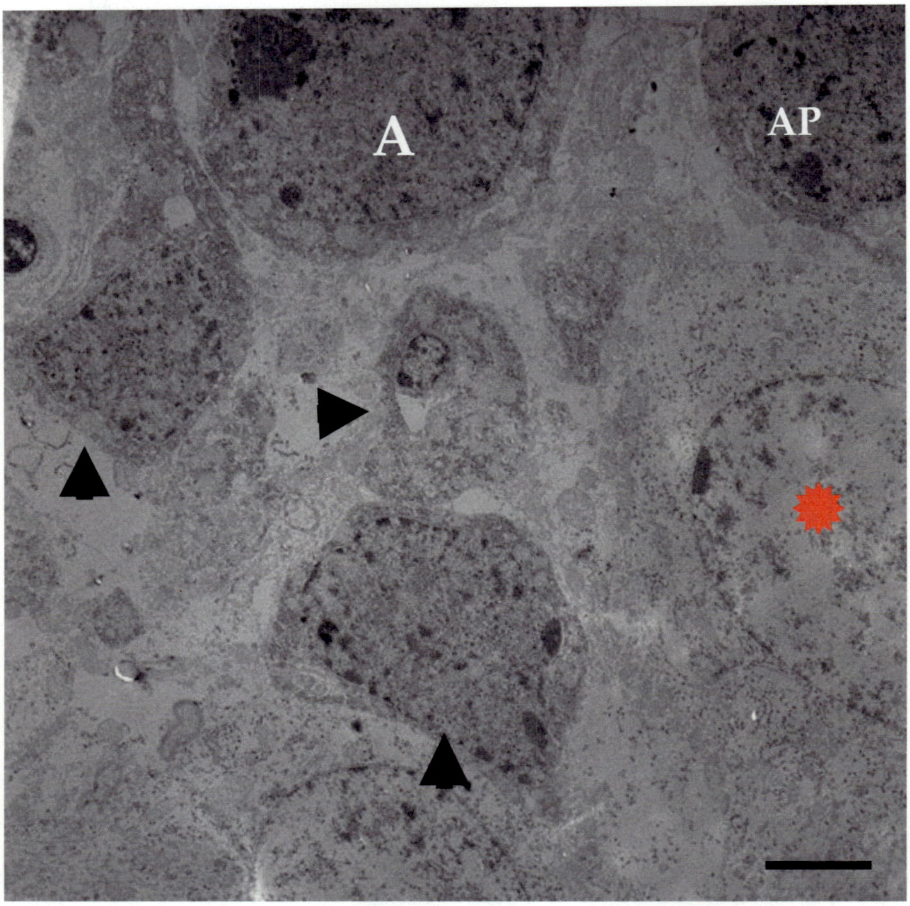

Figure 14. Control group: apoptic neurons(AP) are seen with chromatin margination and clumping. Apoptotic like bodies (arrowheads). Right of photograph (star) shows normal neuron. Scale bar 4 μm.

4. Discussion

Dark neurons have been reported in the brain of experimental animals exposed to various pathological conditions. Morphologically DNs are characterized by at least six features namely: hyperbasophilia, argyrophilia, disappearance of antigenicity, ultrastructural compaction, volume reduction and increased electrondensity (31). On the basis of ultrastructural differences four types of dark neurons are descripted: the Huntington type, the artefactual, the reversible, and the irreversible (32). They have been reported in Huntington, epilepsy, SD, hypoglycemia, and also in aging process (28). The result of our study showed that uncontrolled T1DM accelerates the rate of DNs formation in granular later of DG. We could also show that DNs occur in normal condition that implicates the common nature of dark neuron (31, 32). For demonstration of DNs, we used the selective type-III argyrophilia (method of Gallyas). Gallyas' method is based on the reaction between the physical developer and few chemical groups in tissue. The final product of this chemical reaction would be formation of the crystallization nuclei whose enlargement produces the metallic silver grains constituting the microscopic image (31). DNs of both groups have common features like deep hyperbasophilia, dark staining, and neuronal shrinkage. So the reaction of neurons to different paradigms has resulted to a common morphology. DNs are the final product of a Series of physico-chemical reactions initiated from extracellular milieu and propagate into the neuron (33). At present the only proposed explanation for mechanism of formation of dark neurons is the gel concept. In this concept intra neuronal gel constitute a trabecular network surrounded by fluid. Various noxae e.g. free radicals induce release of noncovalent stored energy from gel state and as a results of gel contracture a large volume of cytoplasm contents is pressed out and lead to neuronal compaction and electron density of dark neurons. It seems cytoskeletal network would be essential in these phenomena (33-35). However, it has not been defined as some different aspects of neuronal reactions. For instance some neurons with small mitochondrion size brown grain in their perikarya were noticed. It is believed these types of neurons are in recovering phase (reversible type) in contrast to real dark neuron (dead or irreversible) (36).Interestingly reversible dark neurons were only seen in diabetic group. At present we can't explain why reversible neurons were seen only in diabetic group but the severity of initiating insult, not its nature, may be a determinant. In diabetes more neurons were probably exposed to noxa e, g free radicals but the response of neurons would be selective (36). Studies have documented evidence that imply the role of hyperglycemia and increased oxidative stress in neuronal death (26, 37). Based on our results it can be inferred that neurodegeneration or aging process progresses more quickly in diabetes type1 (39). Although the rate of DNs was not significant in control animals, it may raise traumatic origin of DNs. Perfusion of animals before brains harvesting eliminates traumatic origin of DNs (38) as we did in this study. To reveal the ultrastructural changes, we took advantage of TEM study.TEM study provides clear-cut evidences to differentiate the mode of cell death (40). Morphological study of DNs by TEM showed chromatin changes, darkness, and shrinkage and swelled mitochondria.

The pattern of chromatin in DNs showed some differences as follows :(1) chromatin clumping with electrondense appearance and normal shape of nucleus boundaries (most seen in control animals) (2) dispersed tiny clumped chromatin with relatively dark appearance and crenated outlines of nucleus (3) large clumped irregular chromatin with irregular outlines of nucleus. The last two patterns were only seen in diabetic animals. To the best of our knowledge this diversity in chromatin and nucleus morphology was not discussed in other related researches. Another characteristic of dark neuron was swelled mitochondria. In line with our findings the same characteristics have been reported in dark neurons (41). The same Chromatin changes (condensation and margination), neuronal darkness and shrinkage are considered as the hallmarks of apoptotic death. Although the apoptotic nature of death in DNs has been discounted and reasoned to TUNEL assay, it should be emphasized TUNELassay is based on caspase activity which is not always sole determinant of apoptotic death (40, 42, and 43). Based on our results in TEM, the different nuclear chromatin patterns can be explained in two ways: diverse patterns of chromatin clumping/condensation as a continuum or response of neuronal subtypes e.g. basket cells in granular layer. It seems apoptotic neurons or DNs represents a common way of death with some differences in intracellular pathways. Cell death can be classified into two major categories: apoptosis (with a variety of chromatin changes) and necrosis (40).The mechanism of DNs production that is proposed is gel-gel transition. The gel–gel phase transition is associated with morphological changes in neuron such as shrinkage, which is not seen in necrosis. Apoptotic neurons also undergo a rapid shrinkage. Thus, the mechanism of compaction in apoptotic neurons might involve the gel–gel phase transition (44-46). In conclusion; dark neurons occur naturally in CNS and diabetes mellitus as a metabolic disorder (common nature of dark neurons formation) accelerates dark neurons formation and consequently brain aging. We propose the future studies focus more on the preventive mechanisms of DNs formation in T1DM.

Author details

Shahriar Ahmadpour
Advanced Medical Technology Department, Iranian Applied Research Center for Public Health and Sustainable Development (IRCPHD), North Khorasan University of Medical Sciences, Bojnurd, Iran

5. References

[1] Sima AA F, Kamiya H, Li G J. (2004) Insulin, C-peptide, hyperglycemia, and central nervous system complications in diabetes. Eur J Pharmacol. Apr 19; 490(1-3): 187-97

[2] Tripathi BK, Srivastava AK. (2006) Diabetes mellitus: complications and therapeutics. Med Sci Monit. Jul;12(7):RA130-47.

[3] Miles WR, Root HF . (1922)Psychologic tests applied to diabetic patients. Arch Intern Med:30:767–777

[4] Kamijo M, Cheian P V, Sima AA F. (1993) The preventive effect of aldose reductase inhibition on diabetic optic neuropathy in the BB/W-rat. Diabetologia. Oct; 36(10):893-8.

[5] Mooradian A D . (1997)Central nervous system complications of diabetes mellitus-aPerspective from blood brain barrier.Brain ResRev.; 23:210-18.

[6] Northam EA, Rankins D, Lin A, Wellard RM, Pell GS, Finch SJ,Werther GA, Cameron FJ (2009)Central nervous system function in youth with type 1 diabetes 12 years after disease onset. Diabetes Care; 32:445–450

[7] Garg A, Bonanome A, Grundy SM et al (1988)Comparison of high carbohydrate diet with a high monounsaturated-fat-diet in patients with noninsulin dependent diabetes mellitus. N Engl J Med,; 319: 829–34

[8] Musen G, Lyoo IK, Sparks CR, Weinger K, Hwang J, Ryan CM,Jimerson DC, Hennen J, Renshaw PF, Jacobson AM (2006)Effects of type 1 diabetes on gray matter density as measured byvoxel-based morphometry. Diabetes;55:326–333

[9] Sima AA F, Kamiya H, Li G J.(2004)Insulin, C-peptide, hyperglycemia, and central nervous system complications in diabetes. Eur J Pharmacol. Apr 19; 490(1-3):187-97.

[10] Ott A, Stolk RP, van Harskamp F, Pols HA, Hofman A, Breteler MM. (1999)Diabetes mellitus and the risk of dementia: The Rotterdam Study. Neurology. Dec 10; 53(9):1937-42.

[11] Jason D. Huber, Reyna L. VanGilder, and Kimberly A. Houser. Streptozotocin-induced diabetes progressively increases blood-brain barrierpermeability in specific brain regions in rats. *Am J Physiol Heart Circ Physiol* , 2006;291: 2660–68

[12] Huang TJ, Price SA, Chilton L, Calcutt NA, Tomlinson DR, Verkhratsky A, et al. (2003)Insulin prevents depolarization of the mitochondrial inner membrane in sensory neuronsof type 1 diabetic rats in the presence of sustained hyperglycemia. Diabetes. Aug; 52(8):2129-36.

[13] Okouchi M, Ekshyyan O, Maracine M, Aw TY.(2007)Neuronal apoptosis in neurodegeneration. Antioxid Redox Signal. Aug; 9(8):1059-96.

[14] Aragno M, Mastrocola R, Brignardello E, Catalano M , Robino G, Manti R, et al. (2002)Dehydroepandrestrone modulates nuclear factor-kB activation in hippocampus of diabetic rats. Endocrinol; 143(9): 3250-8.

[15] Aragno M, Mastrocola R, Brignardello E, Catalano M , Robino G, Manti R, et al. (2002)Dehydroepandrestrone modulates nuclear factor-kB activation in hippocampus of diabetic rats. Endocrinol; 143(9): 3250-8.

[16] Witter MP, Amaral DG. 2004. The Rat Nervous System,. 3rd ed. California, USA: Elsevier Academic ;. p: 637-703.

[17] Small SA, Chawla MK, Buonocore M, Rapp PR, Barnes CA. . (2004). Imaging correlates of brain function in monkeys and rats isolates a hippocampal subregion differentially vulnerable to aging. Proc Natl Acad Sci U S AMay 4; 101(18):7181-6.

[18] Lobnig BM, Krömeke O, Optenhostert-Porst C, Wolf OT. (2006)Hippocampal volume and cognitive performance in long-standing Type 1 diabetic patients without macrovascular complications. Diabet Med. Jan; 23(1):32-9.

[19] Saravia FE, Revsin Y, Gonzalez Deniselle MC, Gonzalez SL, Roig P, Lima A, et al.(2002)Increased astrocyte reactivity in the hippocampus of murine models of type 1 diabetes: the nonobese diabetic (NOD) and streptozotocin-treated mice. Brain Res. 13; 957(2):345-53

[20] Stewart MG, Daviies HA, Sandi C, Kraev IV, Rogachevsky VV, Peddie CJ, et al.(2005) Stress suppresses and learning induces plasticity in CA3 of rat hippocampus: a three-dimentional ultrastructtural study of thorny excrescences and their post synaptic densities. Neurosci;131:43-54

[21] MagariñosAM, McEwen BS. (2000) Experimental diabetes in rats causes hippocampal dendritic and synaptic reorganization and increased glucocorticoid reactivity to stress. Proc Natl Acad Sci U S A. 26;97(20):11056

[22] Saravia FE, Revsin Y, Gonzalez Deniselle MC, Gonzalez SL, Roig P, Lima A, et al. (2002) Increased astrocyte reactivity in the hippocampus of murine models of type 1 diabetes: the nonobese diabetic (NOD) and streptozotocin-treated mice. Brain Res. 13; 957(2):345-53

[23] Choi JH, Hwang IK, Yi SS, Yoo KS, Lee CH, Shin HC,Yoon YS, Won MH,(2009)Effects of streptozotocin-induced type 1diabetes on cell proliferation and neuronal differentiation in the dentate gyrus; correlation with memory impairment,Korean J Anat, , 42(1):41–48.

[24] Reagan LP.(2005)Neuronal insulin signal transduction mechanisms in diabetes phenotypes. Neurobiol Aging.;26 Suppl 1:56-9.

[25] Okouchi M, Okayama N, Aw TY. (2005)Differential susceptibility of naive and differentiated PC-12 cells to methylglyoxal-inducedapoptosis: influence of cellular redox. Curr Neurovasc Res.; 2(1):13-22.

[26] Li ZG, Zhang W, Grunberger G, Sima AA. (2002)Hippocampal neuronal apoptosis in type 1 diabetes. Brain Res. 16; 946(2):221-31

[27] Ahmadpour sh, Sadegi Y, sheibanifar M, Haghir H (2010)Neuronal death in dentate gyrus and CA3 in diabetic rats: effects of insulin and ascorbic acid .Journal of Hormozan medical sciences, 13(4).

[28] Ahmadpour sh, Sadegi Y,Haghir H. (2010)Streptozotocin-induced hyperglycemia produces dark neuron in CA3 region of hippocampus in rats AJMS ., 1(2):11-15

[29] Ahmadpour sh, Haghir H. (2011)Diabetes mellitus type1 induces dark neuron formation in the dentate gyrus: A study by gallyas' method and Transmission Electron Microscopy Rom J Morphol Embryol, 52(2):575–579

[30] Piotrowski P. (2003)Are experimental models useful for analysis of pathogenesis of changes in central nervous system in human diabetes? Folia Neuropathol.; 41(3):167-74

[31] Ates O, Cayli SR, Yucel N, Altinoz E, Kocak A, Durak MA, et al.(2007) Central nervous system protection by resveratrol in streptozotocin-induced diabetic rats. J Clin Neurosci. Mar;14(3):256-60
[32] Gallyas F. (1982)Physico-chemical mechanism of the argyrophil III reaction. Histochemistry.;74(3):409-21
[33] Graeber MB , Blakemore WF, Kreutzberg GW. (2002)Cellular pathology of the central nervous system. In:Graham DI, lantos PL(eds).Greenfield 's Neuropathology. Vol.1. London: Arnold Press;.p.123-9
[34] Kellermayer R, Zsombok A, Auer T, Gallyas F. (2006)Electrically induced gel-to-gel phase-transition in neurons. Cell Biol Int.;30(2):175-82.
[35] Kovacs B,Bokovics P,Gallyas F(2007).Morphological effects of transcardially perfused sodium dodcylsulfste on the rat brain.Biol Cell.;99(8):425-32
[36] GallyasF,Zoltany G,Dames W. (1992)formation of'dark' argyrophilic neurons of various origin proceeds with a common mechanisms of biophysical nature.Acta Neuropathol; 83:83:504-09
[37] Csordás A, Mázló M, Gallyas F, (2003) Recovery versus death of"dark" (compacted) neurons in non-impaired parenchymal environment: light and electron microscopic observations,Acta Neuropathol, 106(1):37–49.
[38] Sreemantula S, Kilari E K,Vardhan A V, Jaladi R. (2005)influence of antioxidant (L-ascorbic acid) on tolbutamide induced hypoglycaemia/anti hyperglycaemia in normal and diabetic rats. BMC Endocrine Disorder.;3:5(1):2.
[39] Kherani SZ, Auer RN, (2008) Pharmacological analysis of the mechanism of dark neuron production in cerebral cortex, Acta Neuropathol, , 116(4):447–452.
[40] Vohra BP, James TJ, Sharma SP, Kansal VK, Chudhary A,Gupta SK, (2002)Dark neurons in the ageing cerebellum: their mode of formation and effect of Maharishi Amrit Kalash,Biogerontology, , 3(6):347–354.
[41] Nagańska E, Matyja E. (2001) Ultrastructural characteristics of necrotic and apoptotic mode of neuronal cell death in a model of anoxia in vitro. Folia Neuropathol. 39(3):129-39
[42] Gallyas F, Kiglics V, Baracskay P, Juhász G, Czurkó A, (2008) The mode of death of epilepsy-induced "dark" neurons is neither necrosis nor apoptosis: an electron-microscopicstudy, Brain Res, 1239:207–215.
[43] Bröker LE, Kruyt FA, Giaccone G, (2005) Cell death independent of caspases: a review, Clin Cancer Res 11(9):3155–3162.
[44] Yardimoglu M, Ilbay G, Kokturk S, Onar FD, Sahin D,Alkan F, Dalcik H, (2007)Light and electron microscopic examinations in the hippocampus of the rat brain following PTZ-induced epileptic seizures, JABS Journal of Applied Biological Sciences1(3):97–106.
[45] Gallyas F, Csordás A, Schwarcz A, Mázló M, (2005) "Dark"(compacted) neurons may not die through the necrotic pathway, Exp Brain Res 160(4):473–486.

[46] Rello S, Stockert JC, Moreno V, Gámez A, Pacheco M,Juarranz A, Cañete M, Villanueva A, (2005) Morphological criteria to distinguish cell death induced by apoptotic and necrotic treatments, Apoptosis10(1):201–208.

[47] Pollack GH, (1996)Phase transitions and the molecular mechanism of contraction, Biophys Chem, 59(3):315–328.

Chapter 2

Bio-Chemical Aspects, Pathophysiology of Microalbuminuria and Glycated Hemoglobin in Type 2 Diabetes Mellitus

Manjunatha B. K. Goud, Sarsina O. Devi,
Bhavna Nayal and Saidunnisa Begum

Additional information is available at the end of the chapter

http://dx.doi.org/10.5772/50398

1. Introduction

Diabetes mellitus is a chronic metabolic disorder characterized by hyperglycemia and derangement in protein and fat metabolism [1]. The worldwide prevalence of diabetes was approximately 2.8% in 2000 and is estimated to grow to 4.4% by 2030. Approximately 40% of patients with type 1 diabetes and 5 - 15% of patients with type 2 diabetes eventually develop end stage renal disease (ESRD), although the incidence is substantially higher in certain ethnic groups [2, 3]. The main risk factors for the development of diabetes are ethnic variations, changes in the food habits, obesity and altered lifestyles. However in type 2 diabetic patient additional factors, related or unrelated to diabetes plays an important role in causation of diabetic nephropathy such as hypertension, dyslipidemia, obesity and it has been named as metabolic syndrome [4]. There are mainly three types of diabetes which include Type 1 diabetes, Type 2 diabetes including a related condition called pre-diabetes and gestational diabetes. The occurrence of diabetic nephropathy varies with type of diabetes and highest risk indiviusuals are type 1 diabetics, but also type 2 diabetics have significant risk. The studies have shown that incidence of renal failure in type 1diabetes may be decreasing due to better preventive measures. However the incidence of renal complications in type 2 diabetes showed uprising [5-8] because type 2 diabetes accounts for at least 90% of all patients with diabetes. Thereby number of type 2 patients with nephropathy and ESRD exceeds those with type 1 diabetes overall.

Diabetic nephropathy is one of the most serious complication of diabetes and the most common cause of end stage renal disease. Advanced diabetic nephropathy is also the leading cause of glomerulosclerosis and end-stage renal disease worldwide. 20% to 40% of patients with diabetes ultimately develop nephropathy, although the reason why not all patients with diabetes develop this complication is unknown [9]. The combination of hypertension and diabetes is an especially dangerous clinical situation; both are risk factors as singly or in combination for micro vascular and macro vascular complications of diabetes and for diabetes-related mortality. It's unfortunate that most of diabetics at the time of diagnosis will have hypertension and studies have shown that 50% of patients with diabetes and hypertension results in a sevenfold increase in mortality [10]. Concomitant nephropathy in patients with diabetes and hypertension results in a 37-fold increase in mortality.

The main treatment dialysis and renal transplantation are costly [11, 12] and most of the poor patients cannot afford the same. Patients with type 2 diabetes undergoing maintenance dialysis require significantly higher financial resources than those suffering from nondiabetic end-stage renal diseases. Furthermore, this group of patients has a very poor prognosis on maintenance dialysis owing to extremely high mortality due to various cardiovascular events [13].

Is the diabetic nephropathy preventable, the answer is yes as diabetic nephropathy progresses from subclinical disease, through the earliest clinically detectable stage characterized by microalbuminuria i.e., urinary albumin 30 to 300mg/day to overt nephropathy with macroalbuminuria [14-16].The combination of strict glycemic control and various biochemical parameters in the form of microalbuminuria, glycated hemoglobin have decreased the occurrence of nephropathy.

Various sensitive tests are available to identify patients with renal involvement early in the clinical course and clinicians should have the knowledge about diabetic nephropathy in the form of its onset, prevention, progression, and treatment in their patients.

Detection of microalbuminuria identifies not only individuals who are at risk of developing renal diseases [(17, 18] but also cardiovascular events and death [19] in these patients. Up to 30% of people with newly diagnosed type 2 diabetes will already have abnormally high urine albumin levels I.e. macroalbuminuria which indicates that many may have overt diabetic nephropathy at the time of diagnosis.

Renal disease is strongly linked to heart disease and the presence of microalbuminuria is a predictor of worse outcomes for both in renal and cardiac patients. Microalbuminuria does not directly cause cardiovascular events; it serves as a marker for identifying those who may be at increased risk. Microalbuminuria is caused by glomerular capillary injury and so may be a marker for diffuse endothelial dysfunction. According to Steno hypothesis, albuminuria might reflect a general vascular dysfunction and leakage of albumin and other plasma macromolecules such as low density lipoproteins into the vessel wall that may lead to inflammatory responses and in turn start the atherosclerotic process [20, 21].

Recently, it has been suggested that microalbuminuria may be a risk factor for the development of cardiovascular disease in non-diabetics and may therefore have a role in screening programs [22].

Early detection of nephropathy through screening of diabetic patients allows early intervention and better control of progression of nephropathy and cardiovascular events and mortality.

1.1. Socio-economic burden of diabetes in India

Type 2 diabetes is the commonest form of diabetes constituting 90% of the diabetic population in any country and prevalence of diabetes is estimated to increase from 4% in 1995 to 5.4% by the year 2025 (23). The countries with the largest number of diabetic subjects are India, China and U.S. and in the former two countries diabetes occurs mostly in the age range of 45-64yrs, in contrast with an age of >65 in the developed countries. Epidemiological studies conducted in India showed that not only was the prevalence high in urban India but it was also increasing [24-26]. This is mainly attributed to life style changes and genetic predisposition in Indian population.

The period between1989-95 showed a 40% rise in the prevalence and subsequently a further increase of 16.4% was seen in the next 5 years. A national survey of diabetes conducted in six major cities in India in the year 2000 showed that the prevalence of diabetes in urban adults was 12.1%. The prevalence of impaired glucose tolerance (IGT) was also high (14.0%). A younger age at onset of diabetes had been noted in Asian Indians in several studies [26, 27].

In the national study, onset of diabetes occurred before the age of 50 years in 54.1% of cases, implying that these subjects developed diabetes in the most productive years of their life and had a greater chance of developing the chronic complications of diabetes. The recent studies found that the occurrence of diabetic nephropathy with respect to age is been decreasing and most of people affected in early ages.

Table 1 shows the prevalence of the vascular complications observed in a study by the Diabetes Research Centre [28].

Microvascular		Macrovascular	
Retinopathy	23.7	Cardiovascular disease	11.4
Background	20.0	Peripheral vascular disease	4.0
Proliferative	3.7	Cerebrovascular accidents	0.9
Nephropathy	5.5	Hypertension	38.0
Polyneuropathy	27.5		

Table 1. Prevalence (%) of vascular complications in type 2 diabetes

Prevalence of retinopathy is high among the Indian type 2 diabetic subjects. Another study done in 1996 in South India showed a prevalence of 34.1% of retinopathy [29]. The prevalence of nephropathy in India was less (8.9% in Vellore) [30]. 5.5% in Chennai [28] when compared with the prevalence of 22.3% in Asian Indians in the UK in the study by Samanta et al in 1991[31].

1.2. The main health problems related to diabetes are

Diabetes can have a significant impact on quality of life by increasing risk for a variety of complications mainly long standing. These include:

Chronic complications
Blindness(Mainly cataract and retinopathy)
Renal Disease
Hypertension
Cardiac Disease and Stroke
Amputations
Nervous System Disease
Pregnancy complications

Table 2. Main chronic complications in diabetes

2. Diabetic nephropathy

The abnormal glycemic status of diabetes is closely related to the development of microvascular complications. However, in humans the evidence of a straightforward causal relationship between hyperglycemia and renal disease is less compelling than in animal models. The development of diabetic nephropathy is characterized by a progressive increase in the excretion of albumin, continued increase in blood pressure and decline in glomerular function which later leads to end stage renal failure. The patients with diabetes are more prone for this condition due to associated factors like hyperlipidemia and hypertension. The mortality and morbidity is high and it's mainly due to a cardiovascular event [32, 33].

There are various factors which lead to diabetic nephropathy like biochemical, hormonal, immunological and rheological.

- Biochemical factors include long standing hyperglycemia and glycosylation process [34].
- Studies have shown that growth hormone promotes basement membrane thickening in diabetes [35].
- Both exogenous and endogenous insulin autoantibodies, IAA contributed in basement membrane thickening [36].
- The red blood cell deformity due to glycosylation and fibrin deposition results in altered permeability and hypercoagulability in diabetic patients [37].

2.1. Genetic and ethnic role

Although we know that all patients with diabetes will not develop ESRD this is due to the good glycemic and blood pressure control. In addition to the risks of poor glycemic control and hypertension, a subset of patients may be at greater risk for nephropathy based on inherited factors. Familial clustering of patients with nephropathy may result from similarly poor glycemic or blood pressure control or may have additional independent genetic basis [38, 39].

Diabetic siblings of patients with diabetes and renal disease are five times more likely to develop nephropathy than diabetic siblings of diabetic patients without renal disease. Even this has been proved by histo-pathological studies in twins with type 1 diabetics [40, 41]. Genetic factors may play an important role in diabetic nephropathy and/or may be clustered with genes influencing other cardiovascular diseases. There is ongoing research in identifying genetic loci for diabetic nephropathy susceptibility through genomic screening and candidate gene approaches [42-44]. A recent genome scan for diabetic nephropathy in African Americans identified susceptibility loci on chromosomes 3q, 7p and 18q [45] and in Pima Indians it has been identified on chromosome 7 [46].

Diabetic nephropathy and hypertension are multifactorial disorders resulting from both environmental and genetic factors, which make it complex and difficult to identify at the genetic level what confers susceptibility to diabetic kidney disease. Gene polymorphism play's an important role for example in renin–angiotensin system, nitric oxide (NO), aldose reductase, glucose transporter 1 (GLUT-1), and lipoproteins which are potentially involved in the genetic predisposition to hypertension, vascular reactivity, and insulin resistance [47].

A recent study has shown that the strong association between a polymorphism in the 5′-end of the aldose reductase gene and the development of diabetic nephropathy in type 1 diabetic patients [47].

ESRD is known to be more prevalent in certain ethnic groups—Native Americans, Mexican Americans, and African Americans—than in Caucasian Americans. Certainly, there is reason for special vigilance for early signs of nephropathy in these high-risk populations, whose members presumably have a genetic predisposition to nephropathy.

The factors which contribute for the development of diabetic nephropathy are shown in Table 3.

Metabolic factors	• Advanced glycation end products (AGEs) • Aldose reductase (AR)/ Polyol pathway
Hemodynamic factors	• Angiotensin 2 / renin – angiotensin system (RAS) • Endothelin • Nitric oxide
Intracellular factors	• Diacyglycerol (DAG) – protein kinase C (PKC) pathway
Growth factors and cytokines	• Transforming growth factor β (TGF- β) • Growth hormone (GH) and insulin –like growth • Factors (IGFs) • Vascular endothelial growth factor (VEGF) • Platelet-derived growth factor (PDGF)

Table 3 Factors involved in development of diabetic nephropathy

2.2. Natural history of diabetic nephropathy (Table 3) and renal changes in diabetic nephropathy

Diabetic nephropathy is a spectrum of progressive renal lesions secondary to diabetes mellitus ranging from renal hyper-filtration to end stage renal disease. The earliest clinical evidence of nephropathy is the presence of microalbuminuria. It occurs in 30% of type 1 diabetics 5 to 15 years after diagnosis but may be present at diagnosis in type 2 diabetics as the time of onset of type 2 diabetes is often unknown. The microalbuminuria progresses to overt proteinuria over the next 7 to 10 years. Once overt proteinuria develops, renal function progressively declines and end stage renal disease is reached after about 10 years.

Stage 1	• Glomerular hypertension and hyper filtration • Normoalbuminuria: urinary albumin excretion rate (AER) <20 μg/min • Raised GFR, normal serum creatinine
Stage 2	• "Silent phase" (structural changes on biopsy but no clinical manifestations) • Normoalbuminuria
Stage 3	• Microalbuminuria: AER 20 – 200μg/min • Normal serum creatinine • Increased blood pressure
Stage 4	• Overt "dipstick positive" proteinuria (macroalbuminuria) : AER > 200μg/min • Hypertension • Serum creatinine may be normal Increase in serum creatinine with progression of nephropathy
Stage 5	• End stage renal failure • Requiring dialysis or transplant to maintain life

Adapted from SIGN Guidelines (48)

Table 4. Evolution of diabetic renal disease

Renal changes are characterized by specific renal morphological and functional alterations which include:

- Features of early diabetic changes in the form of glomerular hyper filtration, glomerular and renal hypertrophy, increased urinary albumin excretion (UAER).
- Increased basement membrane thickness (BMT) and mesangial expansion with the accumulation of extracellular matrix (ECM) proteins such as collagen, fibronectin and laminin.
- Advanced diabetic nephropathy is characterized by proteinuria, a decline in renal function, decreasing creatinine clearance, glomerulosclerosis and interstitial fibrosis.

3. Pathophysiology of microalbuminuria

Normal human urine contains only very small quantities of albumin, less than 30 mg of albumin being excreted by healthy adults in 24 hours. The appearance of large amounts of albumin in the urine is a cardinal sign of renal damage, especially glomerular disease, and is not detectable by screening techniques using urinary dipsticks.

Various studies have shown different factors play a role in microalbuminuria. The two important factors plays a role in urinary albumin excretion are trans glomerular passage of albumin and tubular reabsorption. The glomerular and tubular proteinuria can be distinguished by simultaneously measuring the urinary β_2-microglobulin and albumin [49, 50].

Rodicio et.al., in their article has put forward the causes of microalbuminuria in hypertension which is invariably associated with diabetes as follows: -

- Can be a consequence of an augmented intraglomerular capillary pressure.
- Reflects the existence of intrinsic glomerular damage leading to changes in the glomerular barrier filtration.
- May be the result of a tubular dysfunction in normal reabsorption of filtered albumin.
- It may be the renal manifestation of a generalized, genetically conditioned vascular endothelial dysfunction which may therefore link urinary albumin excretion and elevated risk of cardiovascular diseases [51].

3.1. Structural abnormalities seen during increased excretion of albumin

There is a general belief that increased urine albumin excretion in diabetic nephropathy is mostly glomerular in origin. For albumin to appear in the urine it must cross the glomerular filtration barrier, which consists of fenestrated glomerular endothelial cells, the glomerular basement membrane, and glomerular epithelial cell or podocyte.

It has been seen that increased intraglomerular pressure, loss of negatively charged glycosaminoglycan's in the basement membrane and, later, increased basement membrane pore size, all contribute to the albuminuria. The earliest morphological change of diabetic nephropathy is expansion of the mesangial area [52] and is caused by an increase in extracellular matrix deposition and mesangial cell hypertrophy. After a short period of proliferation, mesangial cells exposed to hyperglycemia become arrested in the G1-phase of the cell cycle and is mediated by p27 Kip1, an inhibitor of cyclin-dependent kinases [53, 54].

Hyperglycemia activates the mitogen-activated protein kinases (MAPKs) which lead to a post-transcriptional increase in p27 Kip1 expression [55].

In addition, ANG II further enhances p27 Kip1 induction and blockade of ANG II attenuates high glucose mediated mesangial cell hypertrophy [54]. Thickening of the GBM is progressive over years; both increased extracellular matrix synthesis and impaired removal contribute to GBM thickening.

There is a decrease in the expression of heparin sulphate and the extent of sulphation followed by increase in collagen type IV deposition. The type of collagen expressed in GBM mainly contains α 3, α 4, and α 5 chains and mesangial matrix has α 1 and α 2 of type IV collagen and increased expression is seen in diabetic populations [56, 57].

The recent evidence shows that an alteration in structure and function of podocytes occurs early in diabetic nephropathy. The podocytes which are adhering to GBM through integrin's are altered due to hyperglycemia.

In addition, renal biopsies from Pima Indians showed a broadening in podocyte foot processes and a concomitant reduction in the number of podocytes per glomerulus [58] in type 2 diabetic patients.

The structural abnormalities seen are:

Mesangial expansion	Fibrin cap lesion
Glomerulosclerosis (diffuse, nodular)	
Basement membrane thickening (glomerular and tubular)	Endothelial foam cells
Arteriosclerosis	Tubular atrophy
Capsular drop lesion	Interstitial fibrosis
Interstitial inflammation	Podocyte abnormalities

Table 5. Main structural abnormalities in diabetic nephropathy

3.2. Glomerular and tubular mechanisms

The alterations in glomerular function and tubular reabsorption play an important role in microalbuminuria. The glomeruli receive 25% of cardiac output per day. Of the 70kg of albumin that passes through the kidneys every 24hr, less than 0.01% reaches the glomerular ultra filtrate and hence enters the renal tubules [59, 60, and 61]. Almost all filtered albumin is reabsorbed by proximal tubule via a high affinity, low capacity endocytic mechanism with only 10-30mg/24hour appearing in the urine [62].

The passage of albumin through glomeruli depends on two main factors, charge and size. The negative charge on the glomerular membrane repels the anionic proteins thereby preventing the passage of albumin molecules through glomeruli normally. The loss of glomerular charge selectivity has been found in both diabetics and non-diabetic population with microalbuminuria [63, 64].

Established microscopic abnormalities include thickening of the glomerular basement membrane, accumulation of mesangial matrix, and increase in the numbers of mesangial cells with disease progression there is a close relationship between mesangial expansion and declining glomerular filtration [65].

Mesangial expansion also correlates inversely with capillary filtration surface area, which itself correlates with glomerular filtration rate. Changes in the tubulointerstitium, including thickening of tubular basement membrane, tubular atrophy, interstitial fibrosis and arteriosclerosis, have been well described. Interstitial enlargement correlates with glomerular filtration, albuminuria, and mesangial expansion. It has been suggested that the accumulation of protein in the cytoplasm of proximal tubular cells causes an inflammatory reaction which leads to tubulointerstitial lesions [65]. Similarly, rise in blood pressure plays an important role by altering the fraction of plasma filtered by the glomerulus.

3.3. Changes in endothelial function

Increased systemic capillary permeability has also been linked with microalbuminuria in healthy populations and recent study shows that endothelial dysfunction leads to impaired insulin action as well as to capillary leakage of albumin [67, 68].

Therefore, microalbuminuria may be a marker of generalized vascular disease, as the formation of atherosclerotic thrombi is related to endothelial dysfunction in arteries. Thus in addition to being an early marker of incipient diabetic nephropathy, urinary albumin excretion may represent common pathways for the development of both large and small vessel disease making microalbuminuria as a possible marker for cardiovascular diseases.

3.4. Cellular and molecular mechanisms

Abnormalities of many cellular processes have been described in the kidney cells of experimental and/or human diabetes. Most work so far has been focused on the glomerular endothelial and mesangial cells. Direct effects of hyperglycemia per se (glucose toxicity), glycation, formation of advanced glycation products, increased flux through the polyol and hexosamine pathways have all been implicated in the pathogenesis of diabetic nephropathy.

Recently it has been suggested that the central abnormality linking all of these pathways is oxidative stress, a defect in the mitochondrial electron transport chain resulting in over-production of reactive oxygen molecules which stimulate each of the above pathways [69].

Increased activity of a large number of growth factors has been demonstrated in diabetes [70].

- Transforming growth factor ß-1 and connective tissue growth factor: May be involved in the fibrotic changes seen in mesangium and interstitium.
- Growth hormone and insulin like growth factor-1 (IGF-1) appear to be associated with the glomerular hyper filtration and hypertrophy.
- Vascular endothelial growth factor (Synthesized by the podocyte): Plays a major role in maintaining the fenestrae in glomerular endothelial cells, has pressor effects leading to constriction of the efferent glomerular arterioles.
- Glucose itself also stimulates some signaling molecules, leading to the increased intra glomerular pressure. Several isoforms of protein kinase C, diacyl glycerol, mitogenic kinases, and transcription factors are all activated in diabetic nephropathy.

3.5. Hemodynamic abnormalities

The glomerular hemodynamic changes in the form of hyper filtration and hyper perfusion results in decreased resistance in both afferent and efferent arterioles of the glomerulus. Many diverse factors including prostanoids, nitrogen oxide (NO), atrial natriuretic factor, growth hormone, glucagon, insulin, angiotensin II (ANG II), and others have been implicated as agents causing hyperperfusion and hyper filtration [71].Hyperglycemia itself stimulates the synthesis of angiotensin II, which leads to various hemodynamic changes in the form of trophic, inflammatory and profibrogenic effects.

The vascular endothelial growth factors (VEGFs), and cytokines, such as transforming growth factor β (TGF-β), may mediate hyper filtration by dilatation of the afferent vessels by inhibiting calcium transients [72]. Furthermore, TGF- β increases NO production in early diabetes, probably by up-regulation of endothelial NO synthase (eNOS) mRNA expression and by enhancing arginine resynthesis [72]. Thus, TGF- β could clearly play a role in diabetic vascular dysfunction [74].

The studies have shown that shear stress and mechanical strain causes hemodynamic alterations by inducing the autocrine and/or paracrine release of cytokines and growth factors.

The factors contributed are:

- Renin-angiotensin system
- Vasoactive hormones such as nitric oxide, prostacyclin, Endothelin -1,Urotensin

4. Role of glycated hemoglobin in diabetes

Glycated hemoglobin (HbA1c), a marker of average glycaemia, is a predictor of micro vascular complications in diabetic individuals. However, it is not yet clear whether the HbA1c is an indicator of the risk of the macro vascular complications associated with diabetes mellitus.

HbA1c is the product of non-enzymatic reaction between glucose and free amino groups of hemoglobin. This reaction, called glycosylation, involves lots of other proteins, too and it is the principal mechanism through which glucotoxicity occurs. Other mechanism involved s is: oxidative stress, activation of the polyols pathway, activation of protein kinase-C, endothelial damage, hemodynamic and coagulative changes [75].

HbA1c reflects average plasma glucose over the previous 8 to 12 weeks as the life span of RBC's is 80-120days [76]. It can be performed at any time of the day and does not require any special preparation such as fasting. These properties have made it the preferred test for assessing glycemic control in diabetics. More recently, there has been substantial interest in using it as a diagnostic test for diabetes and as a screening test for persons at high risk of diabetes [77]. The use of HbA1c can avoid the problem of day-to-day variability of glucose values, and importantly it avoids the need for the person to fast and to have preceding dietary preparations. These advantages have implications for early identification and treatment which have been strongly advocated in recent years.

However, HbA_{1c} may be affected by a variety of genetic, hematologic and illness-related factors [78]. The most common important factors worldwide affecting HbA_{1c} levels are hemoglobinopathies (depending on the assay method employed), certain anemia's, and disorders associated with accelerated red cell turnover such as malaria [79].

Long term prospective studies are required in all major ethnic groups to establish more precisely the glucose and HbA1c levels predictive of micro vascular and macro vascular complications. A working group should be established to examine all aspects of HbA1c and glucose measurement methodology.

The diagnosis of diabetes in an asymptomatic person should not be made on the basis of a single abnormal plasma glucose or HbA1c value. At least one additional HbA1c or plasma glucose test result with a value in the diabetic range is required, fasting, a random (casual) sample, or the oral glucose tolerance test (OGTT) report.

The main long term vascular complications are coronary artery disease, stroke, renal failure etc. The measurement of glycosylated hemoglobin (GHb) is one of the well-established means of monitoring glycemic control in patients with diabetes mellitus [80]. In 1968 Bookchin and Gallop subsequently reported that the largest of these minor fractions, designated HbA_{1c}, had a hexose moiety linked to the N-terminus of the β-globin chain [81].The functions of many proteins depend upon post translational modification, hemoglobin is one such protein [82]. Hemoglobin (Hb) is composed of four globin chains and adult hemoglobin (HbA) is the most abundant form in most adults and consists of two α and two β chains. Fetal hemoglobin (HbF), which is predominantly present at birth, consists of two α and two γ chains. HbF is a minor form in normal adults. HbA_2 is minor Hb after birth and consists of two α and two δ chains. The most common Hb variants worldwide in descending order of prevalence are HbS, HbE, HbC and HbD. All of these hemoglobin's have single amino acid substitutions in the β chain. Normal adult hemoglobin consists primarily of hemoglobin's A (90-95%), A2 (2-3%), F (0.5%), A_{Ia} (1.6%), A_{Ib} (0.8%), and A_{Ic} (3-6%). Glycosylated hemoglobin's (GHb) are the minor hemoglobin molecules separable by chromatographic techniques into three major components: A_{Ia}, A_{Ib}, and A_{1c}. Hemoglobin A_I refers to a combination of these three components [83].

Important perspective studies on chronic complications of Diabetes mellitus allowed us to establish with absolute certainty the role of glycosylated hemoglobin (HbA_{1c}) as a marker of evaluation of long term glycemic control in diabetic patients and the strict relationship between the risk for chronic complications and HbA_{1c} levels. Diabetes Control and Complication Trial (DCCT), a great extent study, has demonstrated that the 10% stable reduction in HbA_{1c} determines a 35% risk reduction for retinopathy, a 25- 44% risk reduction for nephropathy and a 30% risk reduction for neuropathy [84].

4.1. Glycosylation process

Glycosylation is a non-enzymatic reaction between free aldehyde group of glucose and free amino groups of proteins. A labile aldiminic adduct (Schiff base) forms at first, then, through a molecular rearrangement, a stable ketoaminic product slowly accumulates.

In the hemoglobin, the preferential glycosylation site is the amino-terminal valine of the β chain of the globin (about 60% of glycosylated globin). Other sites are: lysin 66 and 17 of the β chain, valine 1 of the α chain. The term HbA_{1c} refers to the hemoglobin fraction of the glucose bound stably (ketoamine) to beta terminal of valines.

4.2. Other proteins which undergo glycosylation

Albumin, α_2 macroglobulin, antithrombin III, fibrinogen, ferritin, HDL, LDL, transferrin; all of them are short half-life proteins. The glycosylation process of short half-life proteins stops at the formation of the stable ketoamine adduct.

4.3. Advanced Glycosylation End products (AGE)

The long half-life proteins such as actin, collagen, fibronectin, myelin, nucleoproteins, spectrin, and tubulin can also be glycosylated. These long half-life proteins (myelin and collagen) undergo a complex and irreversible rearrangement process, with the formation of Advanced Glycosylation End products (AGE). AGE form a family with many compounds, only partially identified; they accumulate in the structural proteins modifying the function of them. They bind to specific macrophage receptors inducing a release of hydrolytic enzymes, cytokines and growth factors able to promote the synthesis of fundamental substance and, acting at intracellular level, to determine a damage of the nucleic acids [85, 86].

Three mechanisms have been postulated that explain how hyperglycemia causes tissue damage: nonenzymatic glycosylation that generates advanced glycosylation end products, activation of PKC, and acceleration of the aldose reductase pathway. Oxidative stress seems to be a common to all three pathways.

5. Note on laboratory aspects

5.1. Microalbuminuria estimation

5.1.1. Sample handling

The collection of sample is very important when you are measuring MA. As many factors will alter the value and errors may occur due to improper aseptic precautions, improper storage and handling. After the collection it is preferable to measure on the same day and if urine albumin is not estimated immediately then urine can be stored at 4°C. Alternatively, 2ml of 50 g /L sodium azide can be added per 500ml of urine. Specimens are stable for at least 2 weeks at 4°C and 5 months at -70°C. Freezing samples may decrease albumin but mixing immediately before assay eliminates this effect [87].

Albumin excretion varies with physiological factors like exercise posture, diuresis. Thus samples should not be collected after exercise, in the presence of urinary tract infection, during acute illness, immediately after surgery or after an acute fluid overload.

The following are considered acceptable [88]:

- 24 hour collection is preferred by some centers but this is cumbersome and errors may occur due to improper sample collection and transport.
- Overnight (8 - 12 hour) urine sample collection
- Short term urine collection i.e. 1-2 hour collection (in laboratory or clinic)

- Early morning mid-stream urine sample is usually rather concentrated and using this sample has good correlation between the excretion rate and concentration of albumin.

Many conditions can give a false positive value. Some of these common conditions are shown in table 6:

• Acute hyperglycemia	• Urinary tract infection
• Hypertension- Independently causes microalbuminuria	• Cardiovascular diseases- Independent of diabetes
• Heavy exercise- Due to increased protein catabolism and altered renal circulation	• Febrile condition and Stress
• Contamination with seminal or menstrual fluid- Which has more amount of albumin	

Table 6. Various factors affecting microalbumin estimation

Semi quantitative methods	
	Principle
Micral microalbumin urine test strip	Immunochemical strip test is specific for albumin. Albumin in the sample is bound by soluble conjugate of antibodies and the β-galactosidase enzyme marker. Conjugate-albumin complexes are separated and the β - galactosidase enzyme reacts with a substrate to produce a red dye. The intensity of the color produced is proportional to the albumin concentration in the urine.
Clinitec Microalbumin	The test strip is based on dye binding by albumin method. It uses the high affinity dye bis (3,3′-diiodo- 4, 4′-dih ydroxy-5, 5′-di nitrophenyl)-3,4,5,6-tetrabromosulfonephthalein. At a constant pH, the strip turns blue in the presence of albumin, and color is directly related to albumin concentration in the urine sample.
Quantitative	
Immunoturbidimetry	In this process turbidity is produced by an immune complex reaction. This causes a reduction in the intensity of light as it passes through the solution. Turbidimetry is the measurement of this loss in intensity because of scattering, absorption or reflection of the incident light in the angle/direction of the incident light.

	Most colorimeters and spectrophotometers can measure turbidity with good precision and accuracy. This is the most widely used test as it can be done on most semi auto chemistry analyzers. It can even be done on automated chemistry analyzers.
Nephelometry	This assay is also based on scatter detection but unlike turbidimetry it measures scattered light at 90° to the incident light. The instrument is called a nephelometer. It is more sensitive than turbidimetry.
Radio immunoassay (RIA)	This assay procedure involves competitive binding between radio labelled and unlabelled molecules of antigen to high affinity, specific antibody. The amount of unlabelled antigen present in the specimen is measured by its competitive effect on the labelled antigen for limited antibody sites. It involves the use of radio isotopes like tritium (^{3}H), ^{131}I or ^{125}I as labels. It has high sensitivity and specificity. The sample values are determined by comparison with a calibration curve. The advantages are sensitivity and precision, whereas the disadvantage is short shelf life and radioactivity of the reagents.
Chemiluminescent immunoassay (CLIA)	Chemiluminescence is a chemical reaction that emits energy in the form of light. When used with immunoassay technology, the light produced by the reaction indicates the amount of analyte in a sample. This again is of two types: Luminescent Immunoassay (LIA): Here the labelled and unlabelled antigen competes for the limited binding sites on the labelled antibody. An inverse relationship exists between concentration of labelled antibody bound to the antigen and the unlabelled antigen. Immuno Chemiluminometric assay (ICMA): This is a sandwich assay in which unlabelled antigen is sandwiched between antibody bound to paramagnetic particles and antibody labelled Acridinium ester (AE). A direct relationship exists between the concentration of antigen in the patient sample and the amount of light emitted during oxidation of the AE.

Note: Advantages of both RIA and CLIA are highly sensitivity, specificity and reproducible. Disadvantages are unavailability, cost factor; proper infrastructure needed, radioactive hazards, Government permission for use of radioactive materials is the limiting factors.

Table 7. Methods of estimation [87, 88]

Marker	Type 1 diabetes sample assayed	Type 2 diabetes sample assayed
Glomerular transferrin	Urine	Urine
Fibronectin	Plasma	Urine
Serum laminin P1	-	Serum
Urine laminin P1	Urine	Urine
Type 4 collagen	-	Serum and urine
Heparan sulfate proteoglycan	Urine	-
Tubular proteins beta-2 microglobulin	Urine	Urine and blood
Retinol-binding protein	Urine and serum	Urine
Tamm-Horsfall protein	Urine	-
Alpha1-microglobulin	Urine	Urine
N-acetyl-beta-D-glucoseaminidase	Urine and serum	Urine and serum
Cholinesterase	-	Urine
Gamma-glutamyl transpeptidase	-	Urine
Alanine aminopeptidase	-	Urine
Tubular antigens,brush-border antigen	-	Urine

Table 8. Newer markers of diabetic nephropathy [89]:

6. Methods of estimation of glycated hemoglobin

In the last 20 years improved techniques in laboratory and new electrophoretical, chromatographic and immunological methods available, gave us a greater reliability on results. However the use of different methods, the lack of a common calibration concerning the same method and the variability of instrumentation do not make reproducible results yet in different laboratories. For this reason studies and procedures of standardization are going on [89]. Methods of GHb assays have primarily evolved around three basic methodologies:

1. Based on difference in ionic charge.
2. Based on structural characteristics.
3. Based on chemical reactivity.

The main methods are,

- Cation exchange chromatography
- Affinity chromatography
- High performance liquid chromatography
- Isoelectric focusing
- Radioimmunoassay
- Spectrophotometric assay
- Electrophoresis/Electroendosmosis
- Electrospray mass spectrometry

6.1. Specimen collection

Handling of specimens before the assay is important as short period of hyperglycemia before blood is taken, leads to an acute increase in the formation of aldimine which may increase the concentration of glycosylated hemoglobin by 10-20%--for example, from 9% to 11% of total hemoglobin-thus reducing the reliability of the test as a measure of long term diabetic control.

Blood samples should therefore be treated to remove the aldimine residues before the assay [91]. In measurement of HbA_{1c} the prevalence of the most common hemoglobin variants (HbS, HbC, and HbD) depends on the genetic background of the population being analysed. There are many Hb variants that result in false low HbA_{1c} level in diabetes. More than 700 Hb variants are known and about half of these variants are clinically silent, their presence may falsely interfere with the measurement of HbA_{1c} by HPLC. Hence, the identification of Hb variants is important to avoid inaccurate HbA_{1c} results [92].

Recent reports have shown that the concentration of total glycosylated hemoglobin measured by commonly used methods may change significantly over a period of hours. This reflects the short term fluctuations in glucose concentration. It is now realized that these rapid changes will depend on the synthesis or dissociation of the labile fraction of HbA_{1c}, which is not separable from the stable form of HbA_{1c}, by most routine methods. In most cases, the labile fraction constitutes approximately 10% of the total glycosylated hemoglobin. This may increase to 25% when plasma glucose concentrations are high, as in poor glycemic control.

These day to day variations in glycosylated hemoglobin concentration secondary to changes in serum glucose are negligible in stable diabetics, but are very wide in unstable diabetics and are almost entirely dependent on the prevailing plasma glucose concentration. Thus, during poor glycemic control there will be large swings in plasma glucose levels, a single HbA_{1c} measurement may be misleading as an index of long term control. It would therefore make sense to measure the stable fraction of glycosylated hemoglobin. However, this is not routinely available because most laboratories measure total HbA_1 or HbA_{1c}, which includes both labile and stable components. Therefore, in unstable diabetics, HbA_I measurements should be interpreted in relation to the simultaneous glucose concentration. To minimize the contribution of the labile fraction, glycosylated hemoglobin should be measured when the plasma glucose concentration is within or near the normal range.

Physicians should be aware of the expected variation in HbA_{1c} during conditions such as [93],

- False increases in HbA_{1c} levels may occur in the presence of HbF (Ex: Hereditary persistence of fetal Hb) and other negatively charged hemoglobin's
- HbA_{1c} levels may also be increased in patients with renal insufficiency, caused by hemoglobin carbamylation resulting from condensation of urea with the same site to which glucose attaches.
- Increased HbA_{1c} occurs with advanced malignancy and iron deficiency anemia.
- Increased levels can be seen in people with a longer red blood cell lifespan, such as with Vitamin B_{12} or folate deficiency.
- Splenectomy can result in elevated levels of glycosylated hemoglobin

- False decreases may result when HbS (Ex: Sickle cell disease) or other positively charged variants are present
- Hemolytic anemia and chronic blood loss result in decreased red cell life span and therefore lower glycosylated hemoglobin levels.

6.2. Factors and clinical conditions affecting glycated hemoglobin levels are shown below [78]

Increased glycated hemoglobin	Decreased glycated hemoglobin
• Iron and Vitamin B12 deficiency • Alcoholism • Chronic renal failure decreased intraerythrocyte pH • Increased erythrocyte life span: Splenectomy • Hyperbilirubinemias • Large doses of aspirin • Chronic opiate use	• Administration of erythropoietin, Iron, Vitamin B12, • Reticulocytosis, Chronic liver disease. • Certain hemoglobinopathies, increased intra-erythrocyte pH. • Decreased erythrocyte life span: hemoglobinopathies, splenomegaly, rheumatoid arthritis and drugs such as anti-retrovirals, ribavirin, dapsone therapy. • Hypertriglyceridemia.

Table 9.

6.3. Advantages and disadvantages of various HbA1c assay methods

Method	Advantages	Disadvantages
Ion Exchange Chromatography	• Can inspect chromograms for Hb variants. • Measurements with great precision.	• Variable interference from hemoglobinopathies, HbF and carbamylated Hb but the current ion exchange assays correct for HbF and carbamylated Hb does not interfere.
Boronate Affinity	• Minimal interference from hemoglobinopathies, HbF and carbamylated Hb.	• Measures not only glycation of N-terminal valine on beta chain, but also beta chains glycated at other sites and glycated alpha chains.
Immunoassays	• Not affected by HbE, HbD or carbamylated Hb • Relatively easy to implement under many different formats.	• Affected by hemoglobinopathies with altered amino acids on binding sites.

Table 10.

7. Diagnosis of diabetes, its complications and management

Diabetes screening is recommended for:

- Overweight children
- Overweight adults (BMI greater than 30)
- Adults over age 45
- Family history of diabetes along associated risk factors such smoking, hypertension etc.

The diagnosis of diabetes is mainly done by using Oral Glucose Tolerance Test (OGT) and the values are shown in Table:

NEW CRITERIA FOR DIAGNOSING DIABETES IN ADULTS	NORMAL PLASMA GLUCOSE VALUES FOR ADULTS		
One or more of the following must be present: 1. Fasting plasma glucose level of > 126 mg/dL on at least two separate occasions.	Fasting	Time Zero	< 115 mg/dL (6.4 mM)
2. Random plasma glucose level of > 200 mg/dL with signs and symptoms of diabetes.	After 75g oral glucose load	30 min	< 200 mg/dL (11.1 mM)
		60 min	< 200 mg/dL (11.1 mM)
		90 min	< 200 mg/dL (11.1 mM)
3. Fasting plasma glucose level < 126 mg/dL but 2 hour glucose concentration of > 200 mg/dL during a 75-gram oral glucose tolerance test.		120 min	< 140 mg/dL (7.8 mM)

Table 11.

7.1. Frequency of visits and laboratory testing

The recommended frequency of follow-up is 3-6 months for patients with type 1 diabetes and for type 2 diabetes patients depending on the glycemic status.

Every 3 - 6 months	**Yearly**
• Glycosylated hemoglobin • Electrolytes, BUN and creatinine • Physical examination including foot examination by filament testing (Carville approach)	• TSH • U/A or urine for microalbumin • Complete chemistry panel (lipids, • LFT, electrolytes, BUN & creatinine) • Ophthalmology examination • Podiatry and nutrition

Table 12.

The frequency of laboratory assessment is subject to flexibility, based on clinical judgment, patients' current control of diabetes, and past laboratory values.

Podiatry if any evidence of neuropathy or breakdown of skin integrity, and nutrition, if dietary non-compliance is suspected.

7.2. Microalbumin testing

Type 1: Annual screening for type 1 diabetes should begin at puberty and for those patients who have had the disease for 5 years.

Type 2: Initial testing at diagnosis and thereafter annual screening needed.

Note: Microalbuminuria is urinary albumin excretion between 30-300 mg per day without an alternative explanation (e.g. urinary tract infection, heart failure, exercise in past 48 hours and blood glucose > 200 mg/dL). If no protein is found in a urine analysis, then a 24 hour urine collection for microalbumin or a spot urine albumin-creatinine ratio may be used (abnormal if > 30 mg albumin/ g creatinine) for screening.

7.3. Retinopathy screening

Baseline Screening:

- For patients with type 1 diabetes who are 13 years of age or older and who have had the disease for 5 years, a baseline screening examination is recommended, and yearly thereafter.
- For patients with type 2 diabetes, a baseline screening examination is recommended at the time diagnosis and yearly thereafter.

Diabetic retinopathy is the leading cause of legal blindness among Americans, aged 20-74. It is highly correlated with patient age and duration of diabetes. Visual loss secondary to diabetic retinopathy is largely preventable if screening is universal and appropriate treatment follows screening.

7.4. Vaccines

- Pneumovaz every five years.
- Influenza vaccine annually.

Regular physical activity: Helps in movement of blood glucose into tissues.

7.5. ACE inhibitors

Recommendations:

- All patients who demonstrate microalbuminuria should be prescribed ACE inhibitors to slow the progression of nephropathy whether they are hypertensive or normotensive.
- Patients with type 1 who are hypertensive and do not demonstrate microalbuminuria should be prescribed ACE inhibitors. Such patients usually develop microalbuminuria in concert with hypertension and are best served by controlling blood pressure initially with ACE inhibitors.

- ACE inhibitors should not be used in pregnant women due to the risk of fetal morbidity and mortality.

NOTE:

ACE inhibitors should be titrated as high as the patient tolerates without orthostatic symptoms, hyperkalemia and /or increasing renal insufficiency.

7.6. Oral hypoglycemic drugs and/or insulin therapy needed

Some of the drugs used are,

- Sulphonylureas

First generation	Second generation
Tolbutamide	Glipizide
Tolazamide	Glyburide
Acetohexamide	Glibenclamide
Chlorpropamide	Glimepiride

Table 13.

- **Meglitinides:**Repaglinide, Nateglinide etc
- **Biguanides:** Metformin etc
- Thiazolidinediones: Pioglitazone etc
- **Alpha-glucosidase:** Acarbose, Miglitol etc

7.7. Life style changes such as cessation of smoking is necessary.
7.8. Health education programs should be started.
7.9. Self-monitoring of plasma glucose using glucometer.
7.10. Management of diabetic complications.

8. Conclusion

The most common chronic complication in diabetic patients is ESRD and several factors contribute to the development of renal damage such as genetic factors, hypertension and hyperglycemia.

The suspected cases of diabetic nephropathy will also invariably have diabetic retinopathy and more predisposed for cardiovascular events and mortality. That's why it's very important to prevent the condition then providing treatment. This is possible, as the progression of diabetic nephropathy is slow and can be detected at an early stage. Microalbuminuria is an early indicator of diabetic nephropathy and urine examination for micro albumin is routinely done to detect and monitor the progression of nephropathy. As many factors can interfere with the estimation of micro albumin, it is very important that high standards are maintained while estimating the MA levels. Other than microalbuminuria various newer markers have come, which still have to be studied for their probable role in its prevention of diabetic nephropathy.

Since, early detection of microalbuminuria can help in early diagnosis of diabetic nephropathy, adequate care and precautions has to be taken while estimating it.

9. Further research

Further studies have to be conducted to find better markers for chronic complications. Regular health education programs has to be conducted at an regular intervals, so that patients lead a better life.

Author details

Manjunatha B. K. Goud* and Saidunnisa Begum
Department of Biochemistry, Ras Al Khaimah Medical and Health Sciences, University, Ras Al Khaimah, U.A.E

Sarsina O. Devi
Department of Nursing, Vidya Nursing College, Udupi, Karnataka, India

Bhavna Nayal
Department of Pathology, KMC, Manipal University, Manipal, Karnataka, India

Acknowledgement

The authors are thankful to Dr. Raghuveer CV, Director and Dean, Srinivas Institute of Medical and Health Sciences, Mangalore and Dr. Ullas Kamath, Dean, Melaka Manipal Medical College, Manipal, Karnataka for their support and guidance.

10. References

[1] Aaron & Vinik. Diabetes and macrovascular disease. Journal of diabetes and its complications 2001;16:235-245.

[2] Gaede P, Vedel P, Larsen N, Jensen GV, Parving HH, Pedersen O. Multifactorial intervention and cardiovascular disease in patients with type 2 diabetes. N Engl J Med 2003; 348:383–93.

[3] DeFronzo R. Diabetic nephropathy: etiologic and therapeutic considerations. Diabetes Rev 1995; 3:510-64.

[4] Remuzzi G, Schieppati A, Ruggenenti P. Nephropathy in patients with type 2 diabetes. N Engl J Med 2002;346: 1145–51.

[5] Ismail N, Becker B, Strzelczyk P, Ritz E. Renal disease and hypertension in non-insulin-dependent diabetes mellitus. Kidney Int 1999; 55:1-28.

[6] Bojestig M, Arnqvist H, Hermansson G, Karlberg B, Ludvigsson J. Declining incidence of nephropathy in insulin-dependent diabetes mellitus. N Engl J Med 1994; 330:15-18.

* Corresponding Author

[7] Ritz E, Rychlik I, Miltenberger-Miltenyi G. Optimizing antihypertensive therapy in patients with diabetic nephropathy. J Hypertens 1998; Suppl. 16:S17-22.

[8] Ritz E, Keller C, Bergis K, Strojek K. Pathogenesis and course of renal disease in IDDM/NIDDM: differences and similarities. Am J Hypertens 1997; 10:202-207S.

[9] Makino H, et al. Phenotypic modulation of the mesangium reflected by contractile proteins in diabetes. Diabetes 1996;45:488-95.

[10] MacLeod M, McLay J. Drug treatment of hypertension complicating diabetes mellitus. Drugs 1998; 56:189-202.

[11] Canadian Organ Replacement Registry (CORR).2001 Annal report.Ottawa, ON, Canada: Canadian Institute for Health Information;2001.

[12] Goeree R, Manalich J, Grootendorst P, et al. Cost analysis of dialysis treatments for end –stage renal disease (ESRD). Clin Invest Med 1995;8:455-464.

[13] Parving HH. Diabetic nephropathy: prevention and treatment. Kidney Int 2001;60:2041–55.

[14] Mathiesen ER, Ronn B, Storm B, et al. The natural course of microalbuminuria in insulin-dependent diabetes :a 10- year prospective study. Diabet Med 1995;12:482-487.

[15] Warram JH, Gearin G, Laffel L et al. Effect of duration of type 1 diabetes on thr prevalence of stages of diabetic nephropathy defined by urinary albumin/creatinine ratio. J Am Soc Nephrol 1996;7:930-937.

[16] Lemley KV, Abdulla I, Myers BD et al. Evolution of incipient nephropathy in type 2 diabetes mellitus. Kidney Int 2000;58:1228-1237.

[17] Marre M, Bouhanick B, Berrut G. Microalbuminuria. Curr Opin Nephro Hypertens 1994; 3:558-563.

[18] Gall MA, Hougaard P et al. Risk factors for development of incipient and overt diabetic nephropathy in patients with non-insulin dependent diabetes mellitus: prospective, observational study.BMJ 1994;314:783-788.

[19] Messent JWC, Elliott TG, Hill RD et al. Prognostic significance of microalbuminuria in insulin –dependent diabetes mellitus:a twenty-threeyear follow up study. Kidney Int 1992;41: 836-839.

[20] Wrone EM, Carnethon MR, Panaliappan LP, et al. Association of dietary protein intake and microalbuminuria in healthy adults: Third National Health and Nutrition Examination Survey. Am J Kid Dis 2003; 41: 580-587

[21] Deckert T, Feldt-Rasmussen B, Borch-Johnsen K, et al. Albuminuria reflects widespread vascular damage. The Steno hypothesis. Diabetologia 1989; 32:219-226.

[22] Gerstein HC, Mann JEF et al. The validity of random urine specimen albumin measurement as a screening test for diabetic nephropathy. Yonesi Med J 1999; 1999;40:40-45.

[23] King H, Aubert RE, Herman WH (1998) Global burden of diabetes 1995-2025; Prevalence, numerical estimates and projection. Diabetes Care. 21: 1414-31.

[24] Ramachandran A, Snehalatha C, Daisy Dharmaraj, Viswanathan M. Prevalence of glucose intolerance in Asian Indians. urban rural difference and significance of upper body adiposity. Diabetes Care 1992; 15:1348- 1355.

[25] Ramachandran A, Snehalatha C, Latha E, Vijay V, Viswanathan M. Rising prevalence of NIDDM in urban population in India. Diabetologia 1997; 40: 232-237.

[26] Ramachandran A, Snehalatha C, Kapur A, Vijay V, Mohan V, Das AK, Rao PV, Yajnik CS, Prasanna KS, Nair JD. For the Diabetes Epidemiology Study Group in India (DESI). High prevalence of diabetes and impaired glucose tolerance in India: National Urban Diabetes Survey. Diabetologia 2001; 44: 1094-1101.

[27] Ramaiya KL, Kodali VR, Alberti KGMM. Epidemiology of diabetes in Asians of the Indian Sub continent. Diabetes Metabolism Rev 1990; 6: 125-146.

[28] Ramachandran A, Snehalatha C, Satyavani K, Latha E, Sasikala R, Vijay V. Prevalence of vascular complications and their risk factors in type 2 diabetes. J Assoc Phy India 1999; 47: 1152-1156.

[29] Rema M, Ponnaiya M, Mohan V. Prevalence of retinopathy in non insulin dependent diabetes mellitus at a diabetes centre in Southern India. Diab Res Clin Prac 1996; 34: 29-36.

[30] John L, Sundar Rao PSS, Kanagasabapathy AS. Prevalence of diabetic nephropathy in non-insulin dependent diabetics. Indian J Med Res 1991; 94: 24-29.

[31] Samanta A, Burden AC, Jagger C. A comparison of the clinical features and vascular complications of diabetes between migrant Asians and Caucasians in Leicester, U.K. Diab Res Clin Prac 1991;14: 205-214.

[32] Cooper ME. Pathogenesis, prevention, and treatment of diabetic nephropathy. Lancet 1998;352:213–219.

[33] Alberti KGMM. Problems related to definitions and epidemiology of type 2 DM. Diabetologia 1993; 36:948-984.

[34] Olgemoller B, Schleicher E. Alterations of glomerular proteins in the pathogenesis of diabetic nephropathy. Clin Invest 1993;71:13-19.

[35] Flybjerg A. Growth factors and diabetic complications. Diabet Med 1990;7:387-393.

[36] Raskin P, Posenstock J. The genesis of diabetic susceptibility. In: Alberti KGMM, Zimmer P, Defronzo RA, Keen H. Eds International textbook of diabetes mellitus.2nd eds. Chichester:Wiley;1997.p.1225-1244.

[37] Lowe GDO. Clinicla blood rheology. Boca Raton, FL:CRC Press Inc, 1988.

[38] Krolewski A, Fogarty D, Warram J. Hypertension and nephropathy in diabetes mellitus: what is inherited and what is acquired? Diabetes Res Clin Pract 1998; 39 (Suppl):S1-14.

[39] Strojek K, Grzeszczak W, Ritz E. Risk factors for development of diabetic nephropathy: a review. Nephrol Dial Transplant 1997; 12 (Suppl 2):24-26.

[40] Seaquist E, Goetz F, Rich S, Barbosa J. Familial clustering of diabetic kidney disease: evidence for genetic susceptibility to diabetic nephropathy. N Engl J Med 1989; 320:1161-65.

[41] Fioretto P, Steffes M, Barbosa J, Rich S, Miller M, Mauer M. Is diabetic nephropathy inherited? Studies of glomerular structure in type 1 diabetic sibling pairs. Diabetes 1999; 48:865-69.

[42] Rudofsky Jr G, Isermann B, Schilling T, Schiekofer S, Andrassy M, Schneider JG et al . A 63 bp deletion in the promoter of RAGE correlates with a decreased risk for

nephropathy in patients with type 2 diabetes. Exp Clin Endocrinol Diabetes2004;.112:135–41.
[43] Hansen TK, Tarnow L, Thiel S, Steffensen R, Stehouwer CD, Schalkwijk CG et al. Association between mannose-binding lectin and vascular complications in type 1 diabetes. Diabetes 2004; 53:1570–6.
[44] Susztak K, Sharma K, Schiffer M, McCue P, Ciccone E, Böttinger EP. Genomic strategies for diabetic nephropathy. J Am Soc Nephrol 2003; 14:S271–8.
[45] Bowden DW, Colicigno CJ, Langefeld CD, Sale MM, Williams A, Anderson PJ et al. genome scan for diabetic nephropathy in African Americans. Kidney Int 2004; 66:1517–26.
[46] Imperatore G, Hanson RL, Pettitt DJ. Sib-pair linkage analysis for susceptibility genes for microvascular complications among Pima Indians with type 2 diabetes. Diabetes 1998; 47:821–30.
[47] Marre M. Genetics and the prediction of complications in type 1 diabetes. Diabetes Care 1999; 22(suppl 2):B53–B58.
[48] Scottish Intercollegiate Guidelines Network. SIGN 11: Management of diabetic renal disease – a National Clinical Guideline recommended for use in Scotland. March 1997.
[49] Laterre EC, Heremans JF. Proteins in normal and pathological urine. Basle 1970;45.
[50] Peterson PA., Ervin PE, Bergard JF. Clin Invest 1969; 48: 1189.
[51] Rodicio LJ, Campo C, Ruilope ML. Microalbuminuria in essential hypertension. Kidney Int 1998; 68: 551-54.
[52] Mauer SM, Steffes MW, Ellis EN, Sutherland DER, Brown DM, Goetz FC. Structural-functional relationships in diabetic nephropathy. J Clin Invest 1984; 74:1143–55.
[53] Wolf G, Schroeder R, Ziyadeh FN, Thaiss F, Zahner G, Stahl RAK. High glucose stimulates expression of p27Kip1 in cultured mouse mesangial cells: relationship to hypertrophy. Am J Physiol 1997;.273(Renal Physiol 42):348–56.
[54] Wolf G, Wenzel U, Ziyadeh FN, Stahl RAK. Angiotensin converting-enzyme inhibitor treatment reduces glomerular p16INK4 and p27Kip1 expression in diabetic BBdp rats.
[55] Wolf G, Reinking R, Zahner G, Stahl RAK, Shankland SJ. Erk 1,2 phosphorylates p27Kip1: functional evidence for a role in high glucose-induced hypertrophy of mesangial cells. Diabetologia 2003; 46:1090–9.
[56] Tsilibary EC. Microvascular basement membranes in diabetes mellitus. J Pathol 2003;.200:537–46.
[57] Zeisberg M, Ericksen MB, Hamano Y, Neilson EG, Ziyadeh F, Kalluri R. Differential expression of type IV collagen isoforms in rat glomerular endothelial and mesangial cells. Biochem Biophys Res Commun 2002; 295:401–7.
[58] Pagtalunan ME, Miller PL, Jumping-Eagle S, Nelson RG, Myers BD, Rennke H et al. Podocyte loss and progressive glomerular injury in type II diabetes. J Clin Invest 1997; 99:342–8.
[59] De Wardener HE . The Kidney. Edinburgh: Churchill Livingstone 1985;:49-50.
[60] Waller KV, Ward KM, Maken JD et al. Current concepts in proteinuria. Clin Chem 1989; 35:755-765.

[61] Deen WM, Myers BD, Brenner BM The glomerular barrier to macromolecules: theoretical and experimental considerations. In: Brenner BM, Stein JA,eds. Nephrotic Syndrome. New York: Churchill Livingstone 1982;.8-9.

[62] Park CH, Maack T. Albumin absorption and catabolism by isolated perfused convoluted tubules of the rabbit. J Clin Invest 1984;73:767-777.

[63] Gosling P, Beevers DG. Urinary albumin excretion in the general population. Clin Sci 1989;76:39-42.

[64] West JN, Gosling P, Dimmit SB, Littler WA. Non-diabetic microalbuminuria in clinical practice and its relationship to posture, exercise and blood pressure. Clin Sci 1991;81:373-377.

[65] Osterby R, Parving HH, Hommel E, et al. Glomerular structure and function in diabetic nephropathy. Diabetes 1990; 39:1057-1063.

[66] Gilbert RE, Cooper ME. The tubulo-interstitium in progressive diabetic kidney disease: more than an aftermath of glomerular injury? Kidney Int 1999; 56:1627-1637.

[67] Felt- Raemussen B. Increased transcapillary escape rate of albumin in type 1 diabetic patients with microalbuminuria. Diabetologia 1989; 32:219-226.

[68] Yudkin JS. Hyperinsulinaemia, insulin resistance, microalbuminuria and risk of coronary heart disease. Ann Med 1996;28:433-438.

[69] Brownlee M. Biochemistry and molecular cell biology of diabetic complications. Nature 2001; 414: 813-820.

[70] C Gnudi L, Gruden G, Viberti GC. Pathogenesis of diabetic neprhopathy. IN PICKUP JC & WILLIAMS G (Eds.) Textbook of diabetes. 3rd ed. Oxford, Blackwell Science Ltd 2003.

[71] Hostetter TH. Hyperfiltration and glomerulosclerosis. Semin Nephrol 2003;23:194–9.

[72] Chen S, Wolf G, Ziyadeh FN. The renin-angiotensin system in diabetic nephropathy. Contrib Nephrol 2001;135:212–21.

[73] Sharma K, Deelman L, Madesh M, Kurz B, Ciccone E, Siva S et al. Involvement of transforming growth factor-beta in regulation of calcium transients in diabetic vascular smooth muscle cells. Am J Physiol Renal Physiol 2003;285:F1258–70.

[74] Tsuchida K, Cronin B, Sharma K. Novel aspects of transforming growth factor-beta in diabetic kidney disease. Nephron 2002;92:7–21.

[75] Lorenza Calisti, Simona Tognetti. Measure of glycosylated hemoglobin. Acta Biomed 2005;76; Suppl. 3: 59-62.

[76] Nathan DM, Turgeon H, Regan S. Relationship between glycated hemoglobin ;levels and mean glucose levels overtime. Diabetologia 2007; 50:2239-2244.

[77] International expert committee report on the role of the glycated hemoglobin assay in the diagnosis of diabetes. Diabetes care 2009;32:1327-1334.

[78] Gallagher EJ, Bloomgarden ZT, Le Roith D. Review of glycated hemoglobin in the mangagement of diabetes. Journal of Diabetes 2009;1:9-17.

[79] Roberts WL, De BK, Brown D Et al. Effects of hemoglobin C and S traits on eight glycol hemoglobin methods. Clin Chem 2002; 48:383-385.

[80] Diabetic Control and Complications Trial Research Group. The effect of intensive treatment of diabetes on the development and progression of long term complications in insulin dependent diabetes mellitus. N. Engl J Med 1993; 329:977-986.
[81] Bookchin RM, Gallop PM. Structure of hemoglobin A,c: Nature of the N-terminal ,8 chain blocking group. Biochem Biophys Res Commun 1968; 32:86-93.
[82] Gallop, P. M., and M. A. Paz. Posttranslational protein modifications, with special attention to collagen and elastin. Physiol. Rev 1975; 55:418-487.
[83] Bunn HF, Haney DM, Kamnin S, et al. The biosynthesis of hemoglobin: A Slow glycosylation of hemoglobin in vivo. J Clin Invest 1976; 57: 1652-1659.
[84] Lorenza calisti, Simona tognetti. Measure of glycosylated hemoglobin. Acta Biomed 2005; 76:suppl.3:59-62.
[85] Bunn HF, Gabbay KH, Gallop PM. The glycosylation of hemoglobin: relevance to diabetes mellitus. Science 1978; 200: 21.
[86] Brownlee M, Cerami A, Vlassara H. Advanced products glycosylation and the pathogenesis of diabetic vascular disease. Diabetes/Metabolism Reviews 1988; 4: 437-51.
[87] David BS, Burtis AC, Ashwood RE editors. Tietz text book of clinical chemistry 3rd ed: Philadelphia: Saunders 1999.p 798-801.
[88] Agarwal S, Sandeep KB, Anuradha R, Vasudha K, Chadha KH, Doli P, et al. Microalbuminuria. Clin. Lab Technology 2002; 3(1) : 14-22.
[89] Salah R, Saleh Ben Hamed, Pajica Pavkovic, Zeljko Metelko. Microalbuminuria and Diabetes mellitus. Diabetologia Croatica 2002;31-4.
[90] Little RR, et al. The National glycoemoglobin standardization program: a five year progress report. Clin Chem 2001;47: 1985-992.
[91] Goldstein DE, Peth SB, England JD, Hess RL, Da Costa J. Effects of acute changes in blood glucose on glycated hemoglobin. Diabetes 1980; 29:623-8.
[92] Chandrashekar M , Sultanpur , Deepa K , S.Vijay Kumar. Comprehensive review on hba1c in diagnosis of diabetes mellitus. IJPSRR 2010; 3:119-122.
[93] Amin A, Nanji, Morris R, Pudek. Glycosylated hemoglobins: A review.Can Fam physician 1983; 29:564-568.

Chapter 3

Type 2 Diabetes, Immunity and Cardiovascular Risk: A Complex Relationship

Daniela Pedicino, Ada Francesca Giglio,
Vincenzo Alessandro Galiffa,
Francesco Trotta and Giovanna Liuzzo

Additional information is available at the end of the chapter

http://dx.doi.org/10.5772/50611

1. Introduction

Diabetes mellitus (DM) is a group of metabolic diseases characterized by hyperglycemia resulting from defects in insulin secretion, insulin action, or both. The chronic hyperglycemia of diabetes is associated with long-term damage, dysfunction, and failure of various organs, especially the eyes, kidneys, nerves, heart, and blood vessels (Expert Committee on the Diagnosis and Classification of Diabetes Mellitus, 1997, 2003)

2. Epidemiology

Diabetes is one of the most common chronic diseases in the world. It is thought that more than 360 million persons will be affected by this disease in 2030 (Wild et al., 2004). Prevalence of diabetes is higher in western countries because of the increasing of population age, physical inactivity and obesity, however it is rapidly spreading also in developing countries due to the socio-economic growth with progressive urbanization and changes in lifestyle.

Cardiovascular disease (CVD) in diabetic patients is characterized by microvascular damage, associated with the development of diabetic retinopathy, nephropathy, and neuropathy, and macrovascular complications linked to the accelerated course of atherosclerosis shown in these patients. Coronary heart disease (CHD) remains the principal cause of morbidity and mortality, in association with an increased risk of developing cerebrovascular disease, peripheral vascular disease and heart failure.

3. Classification and pathogenesis (Expert Committee on the Diagnosis and Classification of Diabetes Mellitus, 1997)

DM is classified on the basis of pathogenetic mechanisms leading to hyperglycemia:

- Type 1, due to a virtually complete lack of endogenous pancreatic insulin production caused by an immune-mediated destruction of pancreatic beta cells (Immunomediated Type I diabetes), or by unknown mechanisms (Idiopatic Type I diabetes);
- Type 2, accounting for ~90–95% of diabetic patients. Its complex pathogenesis, resulting from a combination of genetic predisposition, unhealthy diet, physical inactivity, and increasing weight with a central distribution of the adipose tissue leads to insulin resistance and usually relative (rather than absolute) insulin deficiency;
- Other specific types of diabetes, related to genetic defects of insulin secretion and/or action in peripheral tissues, endocrinophaties, or infections;
- Gestational DM.

Immune system and autoimmunity play a pivotal role in the pathogenesis of type 1 diabetes mellitus (T1DM) (Atkinson & Maclaren, 1994), however inflammation may play a crucial intermediary role also in type 2 diabetes mellitus (T2DM) (Mykkänen, 2000) and in the development of its complications, including cardiovascular disease, thus linking it with several coexisting conditions thought to originate through inflammatory mechanisms.

4. Inflammation, diabetes and cardiovascular risk

Epidemiological studies conducted at the end of 1970 described diabetes as a major independent risk factor for cardiovascular disease, causing 2-4 folds increase in cardiovascular risk (Kannel & McGee, 1979). Atherosclerosis is responsible for the 80% of deaths in diabetic patients (Gu K et al., 1998)[7], and diabetes is considered a "coronary disease equivalent", since several studies pointed out that diabetes-associated CV risk is similar to that observed among non-diabetic patients with prior myocardial infarction (MI) (Haffner et al., 1998; Schramm et al., 2008).

Diabetes is associated with an increased risk of MI and affects more than 30% of patients with acute coronary syndromes (ACS) (Fang & Alderman, 2006). Diabetic patients show a worse outcome after ACS events (Malmberg et al., 2000; Murcia et al., 2004), a more complicated course of the disease and a higher incidence of ischemic recurrences (Cantrill et al., 1995; Miettinem et al., 1998; Shindler et al., 2000). Moreover, if undergoing revascularization procedures, they have a worse prognosis than patients without diabetes (Banning et al., 2010; Hlatky et al., 2009).

Several angiographic studies highlighted a greater spread and progression of atherosclerotic disease in diabetes patients. Moreover, histological specimens of atherosclerotic plaques obtained in diabetic patients exhibit larger lipid core, a higher inflammatory cell infiltration and increased neovascularization (Burke et al., 2004; Moreno & Fuster, 2004).

Since the isolated treatment of hyperglycemia has not been associated to a reduction of CV risk in diabetic people, more aggressive primary and secondary prevention measures are needed in these patients (ADVANCE Collaborative Group, 2008; UKPDS Group, 1998).

The early onset and the burden of macroangiopathy in diabetic patients have a multifactorial pathogenesis and are the result of very complex mechanisms including the coexistence of multiple risk factors, such as obesity, hypertension and dyslipidemia. Moreover hyperglycemia, insulin resistance, hyperinsulinemia and the presence of Advanced Glycation End-products (AGE) in plasma and vascular wall are all mechanisms involved in the establishment of a pro-inflammatory state characterized by the activation of inflammatory cells and cytokine production, leading to immune dysregulation and pro-thrombotic state.

On the other hand, inflammation can be considered a common link between these factors, being involved in each step of atherothrombosis, from the formation to the complications of the plaque, and in the metabolic dysregulation characterizing diabetes.

Several studies have demonstrated a correlation between T2DM, inflammation and innate immunity system. These evidences, together with more recent findings on inflammation and immune mechanisms, could pave the way to a new etiopathogenic hypothesis of Metabolic Syndrome and T2DM, firstly proposed by Pickup in 1997 (Pickup, 2004), and suggesting that activation of innate immunity, together with a chronic inflammatory response, could also play a pivotal and early role in *causing* diabetes, instead of being a mere *consequence* of hyperglycemia, hyperinsulinemia and obesity.

Recent evidences have also shown that adaptive immunity and autoreactivity could play a role in the pathogenesis of T2DM and in its complications (Figure 1).

5. Diabetes and innate immunity

5.1. Systemic markers of inflammation

Established T2DM is associated with elevated circulating biomarkers of innate immunity activation, including C-reactive protein (CRP) and interleukin (IL)-6 and these alterations are also present in patients with pre-diabetes and metabolic syndrome. In fact several cross-sectional studies in non-diabetic subjects, in the general population (Festa et al., 2000; Ford, 1999a, 1999b; Frohlich et al., 2000; Hak et al., 2001; Sakkinen et al., 2000; Yudkin et al., 1999; Visser et al., 1999; Weyer et al., 2002)[23-31], or in individuals with impaired glucose tolerance (IGT)/impaired fasting glucose (IFG) (Muller et al. 2002;, 2002b, Sriharan et al., 2002), have confirmed that acute-phase reactants are positively correlated with measures of insulin resistance, plasma insulin concentration, BMI, waist circumference, and circulating triglyceride, and negatively correlated with HDL cholesterol concentration.

Additional cross-sectional studies in newly diagnosed (Temelkova-Kurktschiev et al., 2002) or established T2DM patients (Arnalich et al., 2000; Leinonen et al., 2003; Richarsdon & Tayek, 2002; Rodriguez-Moran & Guerrero-Romero, 1999) have confirmed that acute-phase

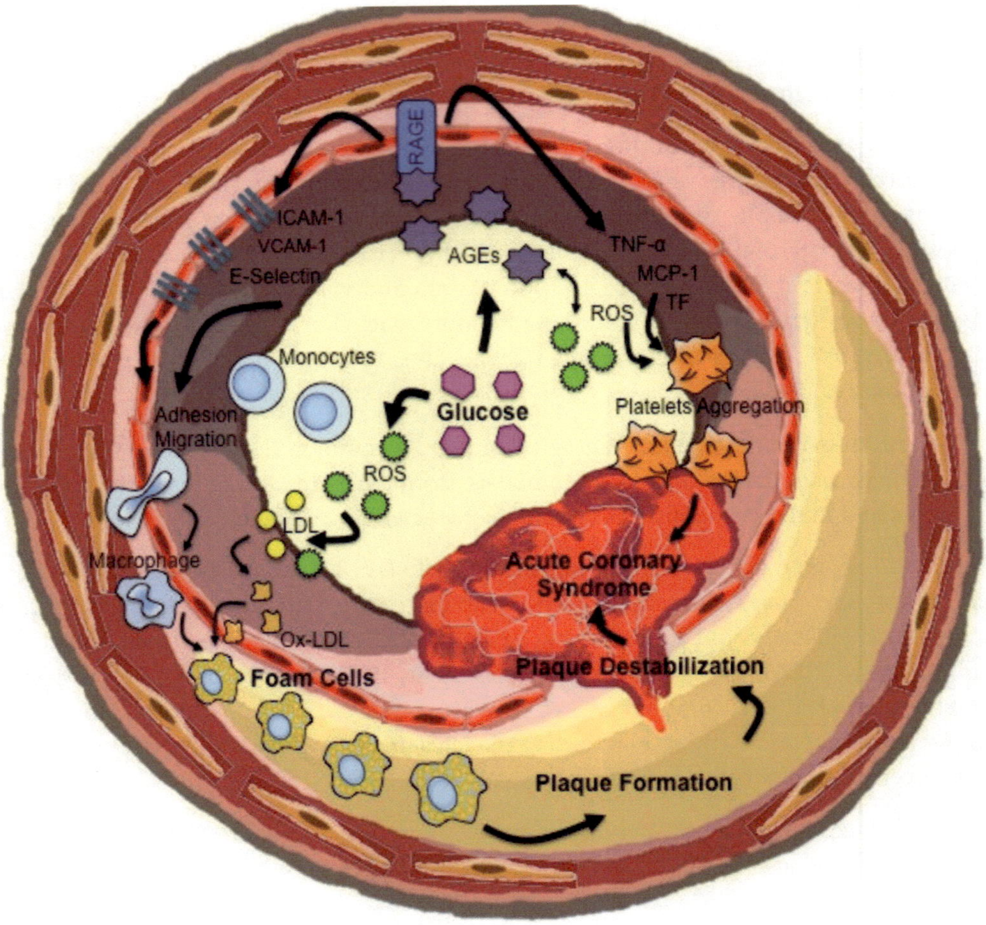

Figure 1. Schematic representation of the principal mechanisms linking diabetes, vascular injury and atherosclerotic disease. Hyperglycemia induces formation of advanced glycation end products (AGEs) that bind to their receptors (RAGE) present on endothelial cells, smooth muscle cells, monocytes and macrophages, thus promoting vascular inflammation, endothelial dysfunction, and prothrombotic state. Hyperglycemia and AGEs also cause generation of reactive oxygen species (ROS), which in turn increase AGE and oxidized low-density lipoproteins (ox-LDL) formation. These pathways are all involved in the development of atherosclerosis and plaque progression/destabilization in diabetic patients.

markers such as CRP and IL-6 are elevated in these subjects compared with non-diabetic controls (Katsuki et al., 1998; Pickup et al., 2000; Winkler et al., 1998).

On the other side it has been shown how abnormal circulating levels of acute-phase reactants, in particular CRP and serum amyloid A, and inflammatory cytokines like IL-6, are good predictor of the development of T2DM in nondiabetic subjects. Schmidt and colleagues (Duncan et al., 1999; Schmidt et al., 1999), using data from the Atherosclerosis Risk in Communities study, showed for the first time that inflammatory markers, such as white blood cell count, low serum albumin, α1-acid glycoprotein, fibrinogen, and sialic acid, predict the development of T2DM and this has been confirmed by several follow-up studies in different populations (Table 1).

Authors	Year	Inflammatory marker(s) analized	Subjects	Follow-up (years)
Pradhan et al.	2001	CRP and IL-6	US women	4
Barzilay et al.	2001	CRP	US men and women	3-4
Vozarova et al.	2002	White blood count	Pima Indians	5,5
Festa et al.	2002	CRP, fibrinogen, and PAI-1	Multiethnic subjects	5
Freeman et al.	2002	CRP	Scottish men	5
Ford et al.	2002	White blood count	US men and women	20
Nakanishi et al.	2002	White blood count	Japanese men	6
Snijder et al.	2001	CRP	Dutch men and women	6
Spranger et al.	2003	IL-6, with additional risk of IL-6 and IL-1 combined	German men and women	2.3
Thorand et al.	2003	CRP	German middle-aged men and women	7.2

Legend: CRP, C-reactive protein; IL, interleukin; PAI, plasminogen activator inhibitor.

Table 1. Inflammatory markers and the prediction of T2DM development

The association between altered levels of acute-phase reactants and the development of diabetes is generally independent of age, sex, blood glucose concentration, family history of diabetes, physical activity, smoking, and baseline atherosclerosis, while it seems to be weaker if adjusted for obesity (Pickup, 2004).

It has been shown that treatment with high doses of aspirin is associated with a 25% reduction in fasting plasma glucose, a 50% reduction in triglycerides and a 15% decrease of total cholesterol and CRP, even if no change in body weight occurs (Hundal et al., 2002).

Recent studies have shown a role played by genetic variations in influencing the innate immune response and the risk of developing T2DM, obesity and atherosclerosis (Fernandez-Real & Pickup, 2008). These variations can relate to genes encoding proteins like inflammatory markers, cytokines and cellular pattern-recognition receptors (PRR).

Genetic predisposition to high transcription rate of TNF-α and IL-6 genes is associated with an increased risk of developing obesity, insulin-resistance and diabetes (Fernandez-Real & Ricart, 2003).

Increased levels of inflammatory markers and insulin resistance have been also connected to a genetically determined reduction of serum levels of soluble CD14, a molecule expressed by macrophages able to bind lipopolysaccharide (LPS), and Bactericidal and Permeability Increasing protein (BPI), produced by neutrophils (Fernandez-Real et al., 2003; Gubern, 2006).

Moreover, decreased levels of mannose-binding lectine (MBL), a protein involved in the clearance of infectious pathogens through the induction of complement activation and macrophage phagocytosis, have been associated both with a raised risk of infections (Summerfield et al., 1997), CHD (Best et al., 2004), obesity and insulin resistance (Fernandez-Real et al, 2006).

5.2. Toll like receptors as link between inflammation and metabolic diseases

Mechanisms by which the activation of the innate immunity can cause insulin resistance have been clarified recently; many studies have revealed how TNF-α could activate the c-Jun NH2-terminal kinase, a stress-induced kinase which serinephosphorylates many signaling proteins, including insulin receptor substrate (IRS)-1 and IRS-2, thereby inhibiting insulin signaling (Morris et al., 2003).

A crucial role, in this setting, is probably played by Toll-like receptors (TLR). TLR are key receptors of innate immunity recognizing a huge number of molecules usually expressed by pathogen microorganisms but absent in mammal tissues, named pathogen-associated molecular patterns (PAMPs), and other molecules called damage-activated molecular patterns (DAMPs); therefore TLR belong to the family of PRR (Kawai & Akira, 2010).

To date, 13 TLRs have been described, both located on the extracellular surface or in the intracellular compartment (Takeda & Akira, 2004). Among them, TLR2 and TLR4 have been associated with metabolic disorders, as well as with atherosclerosis and its clinical manifestations. TLR2 and TLR4 loss-of-function, absence or inhibition in high-fat diet murine models has been related to a decrease in weight gain, insulin resistance and beta-cells dysfunction (Caricilli et al., 2008; Ehses et al., 2010; Tsukumo et al., 2007). TLR4 is highly conserved and selectively activated by lipopolysaccharides (LPS), a constituent of Gram-negative bacterial cell-wall (Kawai & Akira, 2010). Some authors have demonstrated how the lauric acid, a medium-chain fatty acid (FA) component of LPS, trigger TLR4 signaling in macrophages and have revealed how saturated FAs, but not unsaturated, activate inflammatory signals in adipose cells and macrophages (Lee et al., 2001, 2003). Other studies have proposed that the sphingolipid ceramide, synthesized from FAs, might represent a possible link between high-fat diet intake and TLR pathways. Indeed, sphingolipid ceramide is able to activate TLR4 signaling (Fischer et al., 2007; Schwartz et al, 2010), and the inibition of its biosynthesis improves glucose tolerance in murine models

(Holland et al., 2007). However, the previously described studies have not adequately eliminated potential contamination of the reagents used in the experimental condition with bacterial products. Therefore, the direct stimulation of TLRs in various cell types attributed to saturated FAs might be due to LPS contamination (Erridge & Samani, 2009).

The expression in the vessel wall of both TLR2 and TLR4 has a synergistic effect on the progression of atherosclerotic plaque (Monaco et al., 2009; Shinoara et al., 2007). TLR4, whose endogenous ligand is ox-LDL (Xu et al., 2001), is highly expressed in SMC of atherosclerotic vessels, where it has been associated with the induction of a pro-inflammatory phenotype (Loppnow et al., 2008; Otsui et al., 2007). Furthermore, TLR4 has been found in atherosclerotic lesions and at the site of plaque rupture in patients with MI (Ishikawa et al., 2008), and its expression is increased in thrombi from patients with acute coronary syndromes (Wyss et al., 2010; Yonekawa et al., 2011). Moreover, several studies showed that circulating monocytes of patients with atherosclerotic disease exhibit higher expression of TLR2 and TLR4 as compared to healthy individuals (Geng et al., 2006; Kuwahata et al., 2010; Mizoguchi et al., 2007; Shiraki et al., 2006), and an enhanced TLR signaling has been demonstrated in monocytes of patients with ACS (Ashida et al., 2005; Methe et al., 2005; Versteeg et al., 2008).

To date, the mechanisms linking high-fat diets with TLR-signaling and associated pathologies, such as atherosclerosis and insulin resistance, remain to be discovered. As an alternative TLR-dependent mechanism, currently under investigation, the large quantities of lipopeptide and LPS derived from the commensal organisms of the mammalian intestine may contribute to systemic stimulation of TLR2 or TLR4 signaling. Administration of LPS in mice has been associated with an increase of hepatic insulin resistance and a decrease of glucose tolerance (Arkan et al., 2005; Cani et al., 2007). It has been shown that blood levels of LPS are higher in T2DM patients than in healthy controls and correlate with insulin levels and glucose (Al-Attas et al., 2009; Creely et al., 2007; Harte et al., 2010). Hence, an increased level of PAMPs like LPS may play an important role in the development of the inflammatory status characterizing metabolic diseases like T2DM.

Main sources of PAMPs are represented by infections, commensals and diet (Erridge, 2011). It's difficult to assess the quantitative contribution of each of them to PAMPs burden in humans, but increasing evidences are demonstrating that, under certain conditions like high fat meals, PAMPs derived from commensals and diet can effectively translocate from the intestinal lumen to the circulation (Erridge et al, 2007; Laugerette et al., 2010). Indeed, it has been widely demonstrated that oral microorganisms and human periodontitis are associated with an increased risk of developing atherosclerosis and T2DM (Bahekar et al., 2007). The small intestine seems to be the main contributor of the global circulating PAMPs burden, mostly due to the absorption of PAMPs swallowed from the oral cavity. This is probably due to the bigger surface area compared to large intestine and the fat-soluble nature of PAMPs such as LPS, accounting for their easier absorption in chylomicrons with dietary fat, a process taking place only in the small intestine (Ghoshal et al., 2009). Moreover, it is reasonable that the most part of PAMPs absorbed in the large intestine firstly reach liver through the portal system, being there effectively removed from circulation; on the other hand, PAMPs from the small intestine, through chylomicrons absorption, can reach lymphatic system and general circulation bypassing the liver. Finally a quote of PAMPs may come from diet. Interestingly, it has been demonstrated that PAMPs are nearly absent in fresh food, but they can be copious in a number of processed food typical of Western diet, such as meat and dairy products (Erridge, 2010, 2011).

5.3. Role of inflammasomes in peripheral insulin resistance

Recent studies also highlighted a crucial role of inflammasomes pathways both in insulin production and in insulin sensitivity.

Inflammasomes are group of protein complexes which recognize a diverse set of inflammation-inducing stimuli, including PAMPs, and DAMPs (Strowig et al., 2012). The activation of these complexes lead to the proteolitic activation of caspase-1 and, finally, to the production and release of important pro-inflammatory cytokines such as IL-1β and IL-18 (Davis et al., 2011; Schroder & Tschopp, 2010). The most widely studied inflammasome is the NLRP3 inflammasome, which could be activated by a large variety of signals, included PAMPs, DAMPs and bacterial toxins.

A two-step process is required to induce NLRP3 inflammasome activation. A first priming step is usually mediated by PRRs, such as TLR, or cytokines receptors known to induce activation of NFkB, and leads to production and intracellular release of inactive forms of NLRP3. A subsequent activation step induces the inflammasome assembly; it starts in response to a variety of stimuli, such as potassium efflux, extracellular ATP, reactive oxygen species (ROS) and rupture of lysosomal membrane integrity, and leads to caspase-1 activation and cleavage of pro-IL1β. Recent evidences suggest that NLRP3 play a pivotal role both in the early stages and in the chronic progression of T2DM (Kahn et al., 2006). Vandanmagsar et al. found that NLRP3 inflammasome is largely expressed in adipose-tissue-infiltrating macrophages, and it is activated by obesity–associated 'danger–signals', such as the saturated fatty acid palmitate and lipotoxicity–associated ceramide (Vandanmagscar et al., 2011). They also demonstrated how the expression of NLPR3 in the adipose tissue is directly correlated to insulin resistance both in mice and humans and that blockade of NLRP3 could reduce inflammation and improve insulin sensitivity (Vandanmagscar et al., 2011). Other studies demonstrated that during obesity, circulating free fatty acids are scavenged by adipose tissue macrophages to produce ceramide (Shah et al., 2008) and confirmed the role of this lipid molecule in inducing NLRP3 inflammasome activation (Boden & Ceramide, 2008). IL-1β, produced as a result of inflammasome activation, inhibits insulin signaling (Wen et al., 2011) by direct serine phosphorylation of IRS-1 and induces the expression of TNF-α (Strowig et al, 2012), an insulin-resistance-promoting cytokine as discussed above. IL-1β and IL-18 also induce type 1 $CD4^{+}$T-helper cells differentiation in adipose tissue (Vandanmagscar et al., 2011). Moreover, the activation of caspase-1 seems to be related also to adipocytes differentiation and adipokines production (Stienstra et al., 2011).

Inflammasome activation is also involved in impaired insulin secretion associated with overt T2DM. Human β-cells are capable to produce IL-1β when exposed to elevated glucose concentration (Maedler et al., 2002). Several models have been proposed to explain the inflammasome mediated pancreatic islets dysfunction and particularly the role of ROS induced inflammasome activation has been highlighted. Hyperglycemia stimulates mitochondrial ROS production by increasing the activity of the electron transport chain, leading to the activation of NLRP3. Thioredoxin-interacting protein (TXNIP) is usually bound to oxidoreductase thioredoxin, however, when intracellular ROS increase, it seems to act as an upstream specific activating lingand for NLRP3. TXNIP expression is induced by glucose (Oka et al., 2009) and repressed by insulin (Parikh et al., 2007). Moreover, glucose induces the expression of TXNIP in pancreatic islets but not in macrophages(Zhou et al., 2010) and glucose dependent IL-1β secretion in pancreatic islets is inhibited in TXNIP- and NLRP3-knockout mice and antagonized by ROS-blockers. Taken together, these evidences suggest that a chronic condition of high plasmatic glucose levels induces pancreatic islets dysfunction through a mechanisms involving TXNIP-dependent NLRP3 inflammasome and that, once activated, this inflammasome could represent an adjunctive and self-maintaining immune-metabolic stressor.

Hystopathological studies recently showed deposition of islet amyloid polypeptide (IAPP, also known as amylin) in pancreatic islets of T2DM patients (Seino et al., 2001), that seems to be able to specifically activate the NLRP3 inflammasome through a mechanism that involves disruption of the phagolysosomal pathway (Masters et al., 2010).

Additional support for a pathological role of inflammasomes in T2DM comes from human clinical trials in which blockade of IL-1β signaling by Anakinra, a recombinant human IL-1 receptor antagonist (IL-1RA) demonstrated sustained reduction of inflammation, improved glycaemic control and β-cell function in T2DM patients (Dinarello et al., 2010; Larsen et al., 2007).

Moreover inflammatory cytokines such as TNF-α, IL-1β, and IL-6 also downregulate peroxisome proliferator activated receptor-γ (PPAR-γ) expression (Tanaka et al., 1999). PPAR-γ is a ligand-activated transcription factor highly expressed in adipose tissue, where it controls adipocyte differentiation and lipid storage, and modulates insulin action. It represents the target of thiazolidinediones (TZDs) pioglitazone and rosiglitazone, which are demonstrated to improve glycemic control and insulin-sensitivity and to reduce T2DM-associated inflammation (Miyazaki et al., 2001a, 2001b)[120,121].

As noted above, much evidence suggests an intimate relationship among IL-1β, the NLRP3 inflammasome and the metabolism of lipids and carbohydrates. This occurs at the level of enhanced NLRP3 inflammasome activation and processing of IL-1β to the mature cytokine in response to saturated fatty acids and also at the level of glucose metabolism through the requirement of glycolysis for induction of IL-1β mRNA. The pathogenic role of IL-1β in atherosclerotic plaque formation and in insulin resistance in T2DM attests to the importance of inflammasome-mediated pathways as link between inflammation, T2DM and CVD. The exacerbation of NLRP3 inflammasome activation by cholesterol crystals in atherosclerosis (Duewell et al., 2010; Rajamäki et al, 2010) and by IAPP in type 2 diabetes (Masters et al., 2010), provides a positive feedback loop to promote disease pathogenesis.

Taken together, these findings support a crucial role of different molecules and pathways of innate immunity in the complex metabolic imbalance underlining T2DM, and possible contributing to the disease-associated cardiovascular risk. Insight into the above described molecular pathways could help in the design of new therapeutic strategies.

6. Diabetes and adaptive immunity

In the past years, a possible role of adaptive immunity and autoreactive mechanisms in the pathogenesis of T2DM has probably been underestimated and, therefore, poorly investigated. However, increasing evidences support the role of autoimmunity and adaptive immune system in the pathogenesis of T2DM and its vascular complications (Brooks-Worrell & Palmer, 2012; Nikolajczyk et al, 2011). It has been recently demonstrated that T-lymphocytes of patients with T2DM produce large amounts of pro-inflammatory cytokines, such as IL-8, showing in contrast a decreased production of anti-inflammatory cytokines, such as IL-10 (Jagannathan et al., 2010). These functional alterations are consistent with those previously demonstrated in monocytes of T2DM patients (Giulietti et al., 2007; Hatanaka et al., 2006; Pitocco et al., 2009), and result in an imbalance of cytokines network and in a strongly pro-inflammatory environment. High pro-inflammatory cytokines production has been associated in several studies with insulin-resistance and DM development, while the inhibition of some pro-inflammatory mediators prevented insulin-resistance in mice (Arkan et al., 2005; Cai et al., 2005; de Roos et al., 2009; Ehses et al., 2009; Reimers, 1998.

Moreover, the role of a perturbation of T-cell repertoire has been demonstrated in murine models of T2DM. Particularly, regulatory T-cells (Treg) are significantly diminished in the adipose tissue of obese insulin-resistant mice compared to non-obese animals. Treg cells isolated and expanded ex-vivo, in these models, were found able to exert an anti-inflammatory activity and lessen insulin-resistance (Feuerer et al., 2009). On the other hand, Interferon (IFN)-γ-producing cells in the adipose tissue of obese mice may cause an imbalance in glucose homeostasis. The alterations mediated by T-cells with a Th1 phenotype, characterized by IFN- γ production, can be counterbalanced by $CD4^{+}$T-cells with an anti-inflammatory phenotype, such as Treg and Th2 lymphocytes producing IL-10 (Winer et al., 2009), thus underlining the importance of a physiological balance between different T-cells subset in the metabolic homeostasis of adipose tissue, which has a crucial role in the pathogenesis of insulin resistance and T2DM onset. Another cellular type possibly involved in inflammation and insulin-resistance in T2DM are IL-17 producing T-cells, so called Th17. This aggressive, pro-inflammatory T-cell subset has been found at high levels following IL-6 stimulation in the spleen of obese mice, and could contribute to the inflammatory environment strongly related to insulin resistance development and maintenance in T2DM (Winer et al., 2009). Consistently with this hypothesis, high levels of cytokines conditioning T-cell differentiation toward a Th17 phenotype, such as IL-6, IL-1β and Tranforming Growth Factor (TGF)-β, have been measured in diabetic patients (Acosta-Rodriguez et al., 2007; Andriankaja et., 2009; Osborn et al., 2008; Yang et al., 2008). These pro-inflammatory cytokines could promote Th17 cells expansion and inhibit Treg differentiation in T2DM patients. In recent years, a higher percentage of a particular T-cell type, $CD4^+$ $CD28^{null}$ T lymphocytes, has been found in diabetic patients undergoing microvascular complications, e.g. proliferative retinopathy (Canton et al., 2004). An expansion of this particular T-cell population, which is infrequent in healthy young people and slightly expanded in the elderly, has been detected in patients with unstable angina (Liuzzo et al., 1999, 2000); in this population, a percentage of $CD4^+CD28^{null}$ T-cells >4%, representing the 90th percentile of distribution in healthy individuals, is associated with a poor outcome (Liuzzo et al., 2007). These cells have particular aggressive features, showing an increased IFN-γ production and anti-apoptotic factors expression (Liuzzo et al., 2001), and could be involved in abrupt atherosclerotic plaque destabilization through several mechanisms. In fact, $CD4^+CD28^{null}$ T-lymphocytes exert cytolitic effects on endothelial cells and express high levels of TNF-related apoptosis-inducing ligand (TRAIL), thus promoting smooth muscle cells apoptosis within the atherosclerotic plaque (Nakajima et al., 2002; Sato et al., 2006). With these premises, the recent finding of an expansion of $CD4^+$ $CD28^{null}$ T-cells in diabetic patients is extremely interesting, suggesting a possible role of adaptive immune disregulation, either primary or induced by the altered metabolic status and the inflammatory environment characterizing the disease, in the increased cardiovascular risk which is one of the most relevant clinical features of T2DM, accounting for the majority of disease-related mortality and morbidity (Giubilato et al., 2011). Consistently, in the same study $CD4^+$ $CD28^{null}$ T-lymphocytes expansion was closely related to a poor glycaemic control, and was associated with a higher incidence of cardiovascular events during follow-up.

Other fingerprints of adaptive immunity activation have been investigated in T2DM patients.

Increased activity of adenosine-deaminase (ADA) has been described in this population (Prakash et al., 2006). ADA is an enzyme that converts adenosine into inosine through an irreversible deamination reaction, and it is involved in T-cell proliferation and activation (Kather, 1990). Moreover, since adenosine increases glucose uptake into cells, an effect of ADA in reducing tissutal insulin sensitivity has been described (Gorrell et al., 2001). A recent study has confirmed an increased ADA activity in T2DM patients, underlining also an association between enzyme function and fasting glucose levels, as well as HbA1c. Thus, inflammation, T-lymphocytes activation and glucose metabolism seem to be tightly related in the complex setting of T2DM (Lee et al., 2011).

Tregs are another important T-cell type widely involved in autoreactive processes and in the modulation of the inflammatory environment associated with various diseases and pathological conditions. In the setting of diabetes mellitus, Tregs have been extensively investigated both in animal models and human patients with T1DM (Chatenoud et al., 2005, Randolph & Fathman, 2006), while less studies have been performed on Tregs in T2DM. Interestingly, a recent study in mice demonstrated that Treg induction was associated to a reduction of adipose tissue inflammation and insulin resistance, with a concomitant improvement of metabolic parameters of lipid metabolism and glycaemic control (Ilan et al, 2010). Consistently, a subsequent study proved an inverse relation between Treg expression and function and insulin resistance in mice; Treg expansion was also associated with a reduction of signs of diabetes-related end-organ damage, such as nephropathy (Eller et al, 2011).

Finally, B-lymphocytes function has been poorly investigated in T2DM, but some data seem to indicate a role of these cells in the establishment and/or maintenance of a chronic proinflammatory state in this setting. For example, an altered B-cell activity related to cellular TLR dysfunction and leading to increased IL-8 and decreased IL-10 production has been recently demonstrated (Jagannathan et al, 2010).

Overall, these evidences suggest a diabetes-associated alteration of all components of adaptive immunity; these alterations could be implicated in the pathogenesis of the disease and, on the other hand, triggered and maintained by the disease itself, thus creating a pro-inflammatory, pro-atherosclerotic, vascular-damaging environment strongly associated with cardiovascular complications of T2DM.

7. Treating T2DM by targeting immunity

As a role of inflammation has been suggested in the development of diabetes and its vascular complications, TLRs and inflammasome could represent attractive drug targets. Several drugs currently adopted to control hyperglycemia and inflammation and improve prognosis in T2DM patients may also exert their effects on TLR-mediated pathways. For example, it has been shown that statin therapy reduces TLR2 and TLR4 expression (Methe et al., 2005; Niessner et al., 2006; Stoll et al., 2006). The role of PPAR-γ agonists in inhibiting TLR activation both in vitro and in vivo has also been investigated (Dasu et al., 2009; Ji et al., 2009), as well as the ability of some angiotensin receptor blockers to decrease mRNA and protein levels of TLR2 and TLR4 (Dasu et al., 2009). However, although several molecules and drugs could potentially reduce inflammation associated with TLR signaling, studies on humans have to date shown a clear beneficial effect only related to statin therapy. Moreover, no drugs directly targeting TLRs have been developed.

For what concerns inflammasome's related pathways, the role of IL-1β in the impairment of pancreatic β -cell function, leading to apoptosis and decompensated insulin secretion, has prompted the use of anakinra in a double-blind clinical trial in patients with T2DM, that showed an improvement in β -cell secretory function, glycemia and inflammatory markers both during treatment and after drug withdrawal (Larsen et al., 2007, 2009).

A recent study tested in mice the efficacy of a high affinity monoclonal antibody to IL-1β, XOMA 052, showing an inhibition of atherosclerotic plaques formation (Bhaskar et al., 2011). Although clinical trials testing this antibody in T2DM patients failed in demonstrating an improvement in glycemic control, XOMA 052 potentially might reduce cardiovascular risk, since its administration in diabetic patients was associated with a reduction of inflammatory markers and increased levels of high-density lipoprotein.

Furthermore, drugs directly targeting caspase-1 have been tested in mice with promising results in reducing obesity and improving insulin sensitivity (Stienstra et al., 2010).

8. Conclusions

Type 2 diabetes is a complex disease involving the whole metabolic profile of the organism and exerting pathological effects on several organs and systems. The disease is associated with a chronic low-grade inflammation predictive of, and possibly responsible for, many of the clinical signs and complications of T2DM. The diabetes-associated inflammatory status can be the consequence of the metabolic abnormalities characterizing the disease, but increasing evidences are proposing also an important role of immune system disregulation, involving both innate and adaptive immunity, in the pathogenesis of T2DM. Cellular homeostasis is strictly dependent on the cross talk between immune system and metabolic regulators. Hence, any imbalances between them could represent a trigger for metabolic dysfunctions such those related to diabetes. Despite the huge number of evidences at our disposal highlighting the role of TLRs' and inflammasomes' pathways in pancreatic islets dysfunction and T2DM, to date no drugs directly targeting TLRs or the NLRP3 inflammasome have been developed. However, clinical trials have been addressed, with positive results, at evaluating the efficacy of downstream products' blockers, such as Anakinra, a recombinant IL-1RA.

Further studies are warranted in unraveling the complex relationship between T2DM and immune system, and its implication for cardiovascular diseases.

Author details

Daniela Pedicino, Ada Francesca Giglio, Vincenzo Alessandro Galiffa, Francesco Trotta and Giovanna Liuzzo*
Institute of Cardiology, Catholic University, Rome, Italy

9. References

Acosta-Rodriguez EV, Napolitani G, Lanzavecchia A, & Sallusto F. (2007). Interleukins 1beta and 6 but not transforming growth factor-beta are essential for the differentiation of interleukin 17-producing human T helper cells. *Nat. Immunol*, 8, 9, (Sep 2007), 942–949, 1529-2908

ADVANCE Collaborative Group, Patel A, MacMahon S, Chalmers J, Neal B, Billot L, Woodward M, Marre M, Cooper M, Glasziou P, Grobbee D, Hamet P, Harrap S, Heller S, Liu L, Mancia G, Mogensen CE, Pan C, Poulter N, Rodgers A, Williams B, Bompoint S, de Galan BE, Joshi R & Travert F. (2008). Intensive blood-glucose control and cardiovascular outcomes in patients with type 2 diabetes. *N Engl J Med*,358, 24, (Jun 2008), 2560-2572

Al-Attas OS, Al-Daghri NM, Al-Rubeaan K, da Silva NF, Sabico SL, Kumar S, McTernan PG & Harte AL. (2009). Changes in endotoxin levels in T2DM subjects on anti-diabetic therapies. *Cardiovasc Diabetol* , 8, (Apr 2009),20

* Corresponding Author

Andriankaja OM, Barros SP, Moss K, Panagakos FS, DeVizio W, Beck J & Offenbacher S. (2009). Levels of serum interleukin (IL)-6 and gingival crevicular fluid of IL-1beta and prostaglandin E(2) among non-smoking subjects with gingivitis and type 2 diabetes. *J. Periodontol,* 80,2, (Feb 2009),307–316

Arkan MC, Hevener AL, Greten FR, Maeda S, Li ZW, Long JM, Wynshaw-Boris A, Poli G, Olefsky J & Karin M. (2005). IKK-beta links inflammation to obesity induced insulin resistance. *Nat Med,*11,2,(Feb 2005),191–198

Arnalich F, Hernanz A, López-Maderuelo D, Peña JM, Camacho J, Madero R, Vázquez JJ & Montiel C. (2000). Enhanced acute-phase response and oxidative stress in older adults with type II diabetes. *Horm Metab Res,*32,10,(Oct 2000),407–412

Ashida K, Miyazaki K, Takayama E, Tsujimoto H, Ayaori M, Yakushiji T, Iwamoto N, Yonemura A, Isoda K, Mochizuki H, Hiraide H, Kusuhara M & Ohsuzu F. (2005). Characterization of the expression of TLR2 (toll-like receptor 2) and TLR4 on circulating monocytes in coronary artery disease. *J Atheroscler Thromb,*12,1,(2005),53-60

Atkinson MA & Maclaren NK.(1994). The pathogenesis of insulin-dependent diabetes mellitus. *N Engl J Med,* 331, 31, (Nov 1994),1428-3

Bahekar AA, Singh S, Saha S, Molnar J & Arora R. (2007). The prevalence and incidence of coronary heart disease is significantly increased in periodontitis: a meta-analysis. *Am Heart J,*154,5,(Nov 2007),830–837

Banning AP, Westaby S, Morice MC, Kappetein AP, Mohr FW, Berti S, Glauber M, Kellett MA, Kramer RS, Leadley K, Dawkins KD & Serruys PW. (2010). Diabetic and nondiabetic patients with left main and/or 3-vessel coronary artery disease: comparison of outcomes with cardiac surgery and paclitaxel-eluting stents. *J Am Coll Cardiol,* 55,11,(Mar 2010),1067–1075

Barzilay JI, Abraham L, Heckbert SR, Cushman M, Kuller LH, Resnick HE & Tracy RP. (2001). The relation of markers of inflammation to the development of glucose disorders in the elderly: the Cardiovascular Health Study. *Diabetes,* 50,10,(Oct 2001),2384–2389

Best LG, Davidson M, North KE, MacCluer JW, Zhang Y, Lee ET, Howard BV, DeCroo S & Ferrell RE. (2004). Prospective analysis of mannose-binding lectin genotypes and coronary artery disease in American Indians: the Strong Heart Study. *Circulation,*109,4,(Feb 2004),471-475

Bhaskar V, Yin J, Mirza AM, Phan D, Vanegas S, Issafras H, Michelson K, Hunter JJ & Kantak SS. (2011). Monoclonal antibodies targeting IL-1 beta reduce biomarkers of atherosclerosis in vitro and inhibit atherosclerotic plaque formation in Apolipoprotein E-deficient mice. *Atherosclerosis,*216,2, (Jun 2011),313–320

Boden G. (2008). Ceramide: a contributor to insulin resistance or an innocent bystander? *Diabetologia,*51,7,(Jul 2008),1095-1096

Brooks-Worrell B & Palmer JP. (2012). Immunology in the Clinic Review Series; focus on metabolic diseases: development of islet autoimmune disease in type 2 diabetes patients: potential sequelae of chronic inflammation. *Clin Exp Immunol,*167,1,(Jan 2012),40-6

Burke AP, Kolodgie FD, Zieske A, Fowler DR, Weber DK, Varghese PJ, Farb A & Virmani R. (2004). Morphologic findings of coronary atherosclerotic plaques in diabetics: apostmortem study. *Arterioscler Thromb Vasc Biol*,24,7,(Jul 2004),1266-1271

Cai D, Yuan M, Frantz DF, Melendez PA, Hansen L, Lee J & Shoelson SE. (2005). Local and systemic insulin resistance resulting from hepatic activation of IKK-beta and NFkappaB. *Nat. Med*,11,2,(Feb 2005),183–190

Cani PD, Amar J, Iglesias MA, Poggi M, Knauf C, Bastelica D, Neyrinck AM, Fava F, Tuohy KM, Chabo C, Waget A, Delmée E, Cousin B, Sulpice T, Chamontin B, Ferrières J, Tanti JF, Gibson GR, Casteilla L, Delzenne NM, Alessi MC & Burcelin R. (2007). Metabolic endotoxemia initiates obesity and insulin resistance. *Diabetes*,56,7,(Jul 2007),1761–1772

Cantón A, Martinez-Cáceres EM, Hernández C, Espejo C, García-Arumí J & Simó R. (2004). CD4-CD8 and CD28 expression in T cells infiltrating the vitreous fluid in patients with proliferative diabetic retinopathy: a flow cytometric analysis. *Arch Ophthalmol*, 122,5,(May 2004),743–749

Cantrill JA, D'Emanuele A, Dornan TL & Garcia S. (1995). A survey of drug treatment and outcomes in diabetic patients with acute myocardial infarcts. *J Clin Pharm Ther*, 20,4,(Aug 1995),207–213

Caricilli AM, Nascimento PH, Pauli JR, Tsukumo DM, Velloso LA, Carvalheira JB & Saad MJ. (2008). Inhibition of toll-like receptor 2 expression improves insulin sensitivity and signaling in muscle and white adipose tissue of mice fed a high-fat diet. *J Endocrinol*, 199,3,(Dec 2008),399-406

Chatenoud L, Bach JF. (2005). Regulatory T cells in the control of autoimmune diabetes: The case of the NOD mouse. *Int Rev Immunol*,24,3-4,(May-Aug 2005),247–267

Creely SJ, McTernan PG, Kusminski CM, Fisher M, Da Silva NF, Khanolkar M, Evans M, Harte AL & Kumar S. (2007). Lipopolysaccharide activates an innate immune system response in human adipose tissue in obesity and type 2 diabetes. *Am J Physiol Endocrinol Metab*,292,3,(Mar 2007),E740–7

Dasu MR, Riosvelasco AC & Jialal I. (2009). Candesartan inhibits Toll-like receptor expression and activity both in vitro and in vivo. *Atherosclerosis*,202,1,(Jan 2009),76–83

Dasu MR, Park S, Devaraj S & Jialal I. (2009). Pioglitazone inhibits toll-like receptor expression and activity in human monocytes and db/db mice. *Endocrinology*,150,8,(Aug 2009),3457–3464

Davis BK, Wen H & Ting JP. (2011). The inflammasome NLRs in immunity, inflammation, and associated diseases. *Annu. Rev. Immunol*,29,(Apr 2011),707–735

de Roos B, Rungapamestry V, Ross K, Rucklidge G, Reid M, Duncan G, Horgan G, Toomey S, Browne J, Loscher CE, Mills KH & Roche HM. (2009). Attenuation of inflammation and cellular stress-related pathways maintains insulin sensitivity in obese type I interleukin-1 receptor knockout mice on a high-fat diet. *Proteomics*,9,12,(Jun 2009),3244–3256

Dinarello CA, Donath MY & Mandrup-Poulsen T. (2010). Role of IL-1β in type 2 diabetes. *Curr. Opin. Endocrinol. Diabetes Obes*, 17,4,(Aug 2010),314–321

Duewell P, Kono H, Rayner KJ, Sirois CM, Vladimer G, Bauernfeind FG, Abela GS, Franchi L, Nuñez G, Schnurr M, Espevik T, Lien E, Fitzgerald KA, Rock KL,Moore KJ, Wright

SD, Hornung V & Latz E. (2010). NLRP3 inflammasomes are required for atherogenesis and activated by cholesterol crystals. *Nature*,464,7293,(Apr 2010),1357–1361

Duncan BB, Schmidt MI, Offenbacher S, Wu KK, Savage PJ & Heiss G. (1999). Factor VIII and other hemostasis variables are related to incident diabetes in adults: The Atherosclerosis Risk in Communities (ARIC) study. *Diabetes Care*,22,5,(May 1999),767–772

Ehses JA, Lacraz G, Giroix MH, Schmidlin F, Coulaud J, Kassis N, Irminger JC, Kergoat M, Portha B, Homo-Delarche F & Donath MY. (2009). IL-1 antagonism reduces hyperglycemia and tissue inflammation in the type 2 diabetic GK rat. *Proc. Natl. Acad. Sci. USA*,106,33,(Aug 2009),13998–14003

Ehses JA, Meier DT, Wueest S, Rytka J, Boller S, Wielinga PY, Schraenen A, Lemaire K, Debray S, Van Lommel L, Pospisilik JA, Tschopp O, Schultze SM,Malipiero U, Esterbauer H, Ellingsgaard H, Rütti S, Schuit FC, Lutz TA, Böni-Schnetzler M, Konrad D & Donath MY. (2010). Toll-like receptor 2-deficient mice are protected from insulin resistance and beta cell dysfunction induced by a high-fat diet. *Diabetologia*,53,8,(Aug 2010), 1795-1806

Eller K, Kirsch A, Wolf AM, Sopper S, Tagwerker A, Stanzl U, Wolf D, Patsch W, Rosenkranz AR & Eller P. (2011). Potential Role of Regulatory T Cells in Reversing Obesity-Linked Insulin Resistance and Diabetic Nephropathy. *Diabetes*,60,11,(Nov 2011),2954-2962

Erridge C, Attina T, Spickett CM & Webb DJ. (2007). A high-fat meal induces low-grade endotoxemia: evidence of a novel mechanism of postprandial inflammation. *Am J Clin Nutr*,86,5,(Nov 2007),1286–1292

Erridge C, Samani NJ.(2009). Saturated fatty acids do not directly stimulate Toll-like receptor signaling. *Arterioscler Thromb Vasc Biol*,29,11,(Nov 2009),1944–1949

Erridge C. (2011). The capacity of foodstuffs to induce innate immune activation of human monocytes in vitro is dependent on food content of stimulants of Toll like receptors 2 and 4. *Br J Nutr*,105,1,(Jan 2011),15–23

Erridge C. (2011). Accumulation of stimulants of Toll-like receptor (TLR)-2 and TLR4 in meat products stored at 5 degrees C. *J Food Sci* ,76,2,(Mar 2011),H72–9

Erridge C. (2011). Diet, commensals and the intestine as sources of pathogen-associated molecular patterns in atherosclerosis, type 2 diabetes and non-alcoholic fatty liver disease. *Atherosclerosis*,216, 1,(May 2011),1-6

Expert Committee on the Diagnosis and Classification of Diabetes Mellitus. (1997). Report of the Expert Committee on the Diagnosis and Classification of Diabetes Mellitus. *Diabetes Care*,20,7,(Jul 1997),1183–1197

Fang J & Alderman MH. (2006). Impact of the increasing burden of diabetes on acute myocardial infarction in New York City: 1990-2000.*Diabetes*,55,3,(Mar 2006),768-773

Fernández-Real JM & Ricart W. (2003). Insulin resistance and chronic cardiovascular inflammatory syndrome. *Endocr Rev*,24,3,(Jun 2003),278-301

Fernández-Real JM, Broch M, Richart C, Vendrell J, López-Bermejo A & Ricart W. (2003). CD14 monocyte receptor, involved in the inflammatory cascade, and insulin sensitivity. *J. Clin. Endocrinol. Metab*,88,4,(Apr 2003),1780–1784

Fernández-Real JM, Straczkowski M, Vendrell J, Soriguer F, Pérez Del Pulgar S, Gallart L, López-Bermejo A, Kowalska I, Manco M, Cardona F, García-Gil MM,Mingrone G, Richart C, Ricart W & Zorzano A. (2006). Protection from inflammatory disease in insulin resistance: the role of mannan-binding lectin. *Diabetologia*,49,10,(Oct 2006),2402–2411

Fernández-Real JM & Pickup JC. (2008). Innate immunity, insulin resistance and type 2 diabetes. *Trends Endocrinol Metab*,19,1,(Jan 2008),10-6

Festa A, D'Agostino R Jr, Howard G, Mykkänen L, Tracy RP, Haffner SM. (2000). Chronic subclinical inflammation as part of the insulin resistance syndrome: the Insulin Resistance Atherosclerosis Study (IRAS). *Circulation*,102,1,(Jul 2000),42–47

Festa A, D'Agostino R Jr, Tracy RP & Haffner SM; Insulin Resistance Atherosclerosis Study. (2002). Elevated levels of acute-phase proteins and plasminogen activator inhibitor-1 predict the development of type 2 diabetes: the Insulin Resistance Atherosclerosis Study. *Diabetes*,51,4,(Apr 2002),1131– 1137

Feuerer M, Herrero L, Cipolletta D, Naaz A, Wong J, Nayer A, Lee J, Goldfine AB, Benoist C, Shoelson S & Mathis D. (2009). Lean, but not obese, fat is enriched for a unique population of regulatory T cells that affect metabolic parameters. *Nat. Med*,15,8,(Aug 2009),930–939

Fischer H, Ellström P, Ekström K, Gustafsson L, Gustafsson M & Svanborg C. (2007). Ceramide as a TLR4 agonist; a putative signalling intermediate between sphingolipid receptors for microbial ligands and TLR4. *Cell Microbiol*,9,5,(May 2007),1239–1251

Ford,ES & Cogswell,ME (1999). Diabetes and serum ferritin concentration among US adults. *Diabetes Care*, 22, 12, (Dec 1999), 1978–1983

Ford,ES. (1999). Body mass index, diabetes, and C-reactive protein among US adults. *Diabetes Care*,22, 12, (Dec 1999), 1971–1977

Ford,ES. (2002). Leukocyte count, erythrocyte sedimentation rate, and diabetes incidence in a national sample of US adults. *Am J Epidemiol*,155,1,(Jan 2002),57–64

Freeman DJ, Norrie J, Caslake MJ, Gaw A, Ford I, Lowe GD, O'Reilly DS, Packard CJ & Sattar N; West of Scotland Coronary Prevention Study. (2002). C-reactive protein is an independent predictor of risk for the development of diabetes in the West of Scotland Coronary Prevention Study. *Diabetes*,51,5,(May 2002),1596–1600

Fröhlich M, Imhof A, Berg G, Hutchinson WL, Pepys MB, Boeing H, Muche R, Brenner H &Koenig W. (2000). Association between C-reactive protein and features of the metabolic syndrome: a population-based study. *Diabetes Care*,23,12,(Dec 2000),1835–1839

Geng HL, Lu HQ, Zhang LZ, Zhang H, Zhou L, Wang H & Zhong RQ. (2006). Increased expression of Toll like receptor 4 on peripheral-blood mononuclear cells in patients with coronary arteriosclerosis disease. *Clin Exp Immunol*,143,2,(Feb 2006),269-273

Genuth S, Alberti KG, Bennett P, Buse J, Defronzo R, Kahn R, Kitzmiller J, Knowler WC, Lebovitz H, Lernmark A, Nathan D, Palmer J, Rizza R, Saudek C, Shaw J, Steffes M, Stern M, Tuomilehto J &Zimmet P; Expert Committee on the Diagnosis and Classification of Diabetes Mellitus. (2003). Expert Committee on the Diagnosis and Classification of Diabetes Mellitus2, the Expert Committee on the Diagnosis and

Classification of Diabetes Mellitus. Follow-up report on the diagnosis of diabetes mellitus. *Diabetes Care*,26,11,(Nov 2003),3160–3167

Ghoshal S, Witta J, Zhong J, de Villiers W &Eckhardt E. (2009). Chylomicrons promote intestinal absorption of lipopolysaccharides. *J Lipid Res*, 50,1,(Jan 2009),90–97

Giubilato S, Liuzzo G, Brugaletta S, Pitocco D, Graziani F, Smaldone C, Montone RA, Pazzano V, Pedicino D, Biasucci LM, Ghirlanda G & Crea F. (2011). Expansion of CD4+CD28null T-lymphocytes in diabetic patients: exploring new pathogenetic mechanisms of increased cardiovascular risk in diabetes mellitus. *Eur Heart J*,32,10,(May 2011),1214-1226

Giulietti A, van Etten E, Overbergh L, Stoffels K, Bouillon R &Mathieu C. (2007). Monocytes from type 2 diabetic patients have a pro-inflammatory profile. 1,25-Dihydroxyvitamin D(3) works as antiinflammatory. *Diabetes Res. Clin. Pract*,77,1,(Jul 2007),47–57

Gorrell MD, Gysbers V & McCaughan GW. (2001). CD26: a multifunctional integral membrane and secreted protein of activated lymphocytes. *Scand J Immunol*,54,3,(Sep 2001),249-264

Gu K, Cowie CC &Harris MI. (1998). Mortality in adults wit and without diabetes in a national cohort of the U.S population, 1971-1993. *Diabetes Care*,21,7,(Jul 1998),1138-1145

Gubern C, López-Bermejo A, Biarnés J, Vendrell J, Ricart W & Fernández-Real JM. (2006). Natural antibiotics and insulin sensitivity: the role of bactericidal and permeability increasing protein (BPI). *Diabetes*,55,1,(Jan 2006),216–224

Haffner SM, Lehto S, Rönnemaa T, Pyörälä K & Laakso M. (1998). Mortality from coronary heart disease in subjects with type 2 diabetes and in nondiabetic subjects with and without prior myocardial infarction. *N Engl J Med*,339,4,(Jul 1998),229-234

Haffner SM, Mykkänen L, Festa A, Burke JP, Stern MP. (2000). Insulin-resistant prediabetic subjects have more atherogenic risk factors than insulin-sensitive prediabetic subjects: implications for preventing coronary heart disease during the prediabetic state. *Circulation*, 101, 9, (Mar 2000) 975-980

Hak AE, Pols HA, Stehouwer CD, Meijer J, Kiliaan AJ, Hofman A, Breteler MM & Witteman JC. (2001). Markers of inflammation and cellular adhesion molecules in relation to insulin resistance in nondiabetic elderly: the Rotterdam Study. *J Clin Endocr Metab*,86,9,(Sep 2001),4398–4405

Harte AL, da Silva NF, Creely SJ, McGee KC, Billyard T, Youssef-Elabd EM, Tripathi G, Ashour E, Abdalla MS, Sharada HM, Amin AI, Burt AD, Kumar S, Day CP & McTernan PG. (2010). Elevated endotoxin levels in non-alcoholic fatty liver disease. *J Inflamm (Lond)*,30,(Mar 2010),7:15

Hatanaka E, Monteagudo PT, Marrocos MS &Campa A. (2006). Neutrophils and monocytes as potentially important sources of proinflammatory cytokines in diabetes. *Clin Exp Immunol*,146,3,(Dec 2006),443–447

Hlatky MA, Boothroyd DB, Bravata DM, Boersma E, Booth J, Brooks MM, Carrié D, Clayton TC, Danchin N, Flather M, Hamm CW, Hueb WA, Kähler J, Kelsey SF, King SB, Kosinski AS, Lopes N, McDonald KM, Rodriguez A, Serruys P, Sigwart U, Stables RH, Owens DK & Pocock SJ. (2009). Coronary artery bypass surgery compared with percutaneous coronary interventions for multivesseldisease: a collaborative analysis of individual patient data from ten randomized trials. *Lancet*, 373,9670,(Apr 2009),1190–1197

Holland WL, Brozinick JT, Wang LP, Hawkins ED, Sargent KM, Liu Y, Narra K, Hoehn KL, Knotts TA, Siesky A, Nelson DH, Karathanasis SK, Fontenot GK, Birnbaum MJ & Summers SA. (2007). Inhibition of ceramide synthesis ameliorates glucocorticoid-, saturated-fat-, and obesity-induced insulin resistance. *Cell Metab*,5,3,(Mar 2007),167–179

Hundal RS, Petersen KF, Mayerson AB, Randhawa PS, Inzucchi S, Shoelson SE & Shulman GI. (2002). Mechanism by which high-dose aspirin improves glucose metabolism in type 2 diabetes. *J Clin Invest*,109,10,(May 2002),1321-1326

Ilan Y, Maron R, Tukpah AM, Maioli TU, Murugaiyan G, Yang K, Wu HY & Weiner HL. (2010). Induction of regulatory T cells decreases adipose inflammation and alleviates insulin resistance in ob/ob mice. *Proc Natl Acad Sci USA*,107,21,(May 2010),9765-9770

Ishikawa Y, Satoh M, Itoh T, Minami Y, Takahashi Y & Akamura M. (2008). Local expression of toll-like receptor 4 at the site of ruptured plaques in patients with acute myocardial infarction. *Clin Sci*,115,4,(Aug 2008),133–140

Jagannathan M, McDonnell M, Liang Y, Hasturk H, Hetzel J, Rubin D, Kantarci A, Van Dyke TE, Ganley-Leal LM & Nikolajczyk BS. (2010). Toll-like receptors regulate B cell cytokine production in patients with diabetes. *Diabetologia*,53,7,(Jul 2010),1461–1471

Ji Y, Liu J, Wang Z, Liu N &Gou W. (2009). PPARgamma agonist, rosiglitazone, regulates angiotensin II-induced vascular inflammation through the TLR4- dependent signaling pathway. *Lab Invest*,89,8,(Aug 2009),887–902

Kahn SE, Hull RL & Utzschneider KM. (2006). Mechanisms linking obesity to insulin resistance and type 2 diabetes. *Nature*,444,7121,(Dec 2006),840-846

Kannel WB & McGee DL. (1979). Diabetes and cardiovascular disease: the Framingham study. *JAMA*,241,19,(May 1979),2035-2038

Kather,H. (1990). Pathways of purine metabolism in human adipocytes. Further evidence against a role of adenosine as an endogenous regulator of human fat cell function. *J Biol Chem*,265,1,(Jan 1990),96-102

Katsuki A, Sumida Y, Murashima S, Murata K, Takarada Y, Ito K, Fujii M, Tsuchihashi K, Goto H, Nakatani K & Yano Y. (1998). Serum levels of tumor necrosis factor-α are increased in obese patients with noninsulin-dependent diabetes mellitus. *J Clin Endocrinol Metab*,83,3,(Mar 1998),859-862

Kawai T & Akira S. (2010). The role of pattern-recognition receptors in innate immunity: update on Toll-like receptors. *Nat Immunol*,11,5,(May 2010),373-384

Kuwahata S, Fujita S, Orihara K, Hamasaki S, Oba R, Hirai H, Nagata K, Ishida S, Kataoka T, Oketani N, Ichiki H, Iriki Y, Saihara K, Okui H, Ninomiya Y & Tei C. (2010). High expression level of Toll-like receptor 2 on monocytes is an important risk factor for arteriosclerotic disease. *Atherosclerosis*,209,1,(Mar 2010),248-254

Larsen CM, Faulenbach M, Vaag A, Vølund A, Ehses JA, Seifert B, Mandrup-Poulsen T & Donath MY. (2007). Interleukin-1-receptor antagonist in type 2 diabetes mellitus. *N. Engl. J. Med*,356,15,(Apr 2007),1517–1526

Larsen CM, Faulenbach M, Vaag A, Ehses JA, Donath MY & Mandrup-Poulsen T. (2009). Sustained effects of interleukin-1 receptor antagonist treatment in type 2 diabetes. *Diabetes Care*,32,9,(Sept 2009),1663–1668

Laugerette F, Vors C, Géloën A, Chauvin MA, Soulage C, Lambert-Porcheron S, Peretti N, Alligier M, Burcelin R, Laville M, Vidal H & Michalski MC. (2011). Emulsified lipids increase endotoxemia: possible role in early postprandial low-grade inflammation. *J Nutr Biochem*,22,1,(Jan 2011),53–59

Lee JY, Sohn KH, Rhee SH & Hwang D. (2001). Saturated fatty acids, but not unsaturated fatty acids, induce the expression of cyclooxygenase-2 mediated through Toll-like receptor 4. *J Biol Chem*,276,20,(May 2001),16683–16689

Lee JY, Ye J, Gao Z, Youn HS, Lee WH, Zhao L, Sizemore N & Hwang DH. (2003). Reciprocal modulation of Toll-like receptor-4 signaling pathways involving MyD88 and phosphatidylinositol 3- kinase/AKT by saturated and polyunsaturated fatty acids. *J Biol Chem*, 278,39,(Sept 2003),37041–37051

Lee JG, Kang DG, Yu JR, Kim Y, Kim J, Koh G & Lee D. (2011). Changes in Adenosine Deaminase Activity in Patients with Type 2 Diabetes Mellitus and Effect of DPP-4 Inhibitor Treatment on ADA Activity. *Diabetes Metab J*,35,2,(Apr 2011),149-158

Leinonen E, Hurt-Camejo E, Wiklund O, Hultén LM, Hiukka A & Taskinen MR. (2003). Insulin resistance and adiposity correlate with acute-phase reaction and soluble cell adhesion molecules in type 2 diabetes. *Atherosclerosis*,166,2,(Feb 2003),387–394

Liuzzo G, Kopecky SL, Frye RL, O'Fallon WM, Maseri A, Goronzy JJ & Weyand CM. (1999). Perturbation of the T-cell repertoire in patients with unstable angina. *Circulation*,100,21,(Nov 1999),2135-2139

Liuzzo G, Goronzy JJ, Yang H, Kopecky SL, Holmes DR, Frye RL & Weyand CM. (2000). Monoclonal T-cell proliferation and plaque instability in acute coronary syndromes. *Circulation*,101,25,(Jun 2000),2883-2888

Liuzzo G, Vallejo AN, Kopecky SL, Frye RL, Holmes DR, Goronzy JJ & Weyand CM. (2001). Molecular fingerprint of interferon-γ signalling in unstable angina. *Circulation*, 103,11,(Mar 2001),1509-1514

Liuzzo G, Biasucci LM, Trotta G, Brugaletta S, Pinnelli M, Digianuario G, Rizzello V, Rebuzzi AG, Rumi C, Maseri A & Crea F. (2007). Unusual CD4+CD28null T lymphocytes and recurrence of acute coronary events. *J Am Coll Cardiol*,50,15,(Oct 2007),1450-8

Loppnow H, Werdan K & Buerke M. (2008). Vascular cells contribute to atherosclerosis by cytokine and innate immunity-related inflammatory mechanisms. *Innate Immun*,14,2,(Apr 2008),63–87

Maedler K, Sergeev P, Ris F, Oberholzer J, Joller-Jemelka HI, Spinas GA, Kaiser N, Halban PA & Donath MY. (2008). Glucose-induced β cell production of IL-1b contributes to glucotoxicity in human pancreatic islets. *J. Clin. Invest*, 110, 6, (Sep 2002), 851–860

Malmberg K, Yusuf S, Gerstein HC, Brown J, Zhao F, Hunt D, Piegas L, Calvin J, Keltai M & Budaj A. (2000). Impact of diabetes on long-term prognosis in patients with unstable angina and non-Q-Wave myocardial infarction: results of the OASIS (Organization to

Asses Strategies for Ischemic Syndromes) Registry. *Circulation*, 102, 9, (Aug 2000), 1014-1019

Masters SL, Dunne A, Subramanian SL, Hull RL, Tannahill GM, Sharp FA, Becker C, Franchi L, Yoshihara E, Chen Z, Mullooly N, Mielke LA, Harris J, Coll RC, Mills KH, Mok KH, Newsholme P, Nuñez G, Yodoi J, Kahn SE, Lavelle EC & O'Neill LA. (2010). Activation of the NLRP3 inflammasome by islet amyloid polypeptide provides a mechanism for enhanced IL-1β in type 2 diabetes. *Nature Immunol.*, 11, 10, (Oct 2010), 897–904

Methe H, Kim JO, Kofler S, Weis M, Nabauer M & Koglin J. (2005). Expansion of circulating Toll-like receptor 4-positive monocytes in patients with acute coronary syndrome. *Circulation*, 111, 20, (May 2005), 2654-2661

Methe H, Kim JO, Kofler S, Nabauer M & Weis M. (2005). Statins decrease toll-like receptor 4 expression and downstream signaling in human $CD14^+$ monocytes. *Arterioscler Thromb Vasc Biol*, 25, 7, (Jul 2005), 1439–1445

Miettinen H, Lehto S, Salomaa V, Mähönen M, Niemelä M, Haffner SM, Pyörälä K & Tuomilehto J.(1998). Impact of diabetes on mortality after the first myocardial infarction. The FINMONICA Myocardial Infarction Register Study Group. *Diabetes Care*,21,1, (Jan 1998),69-75

Miyazaki Y, Mahankali A, Matsuda M, Glass L, Mahankali S, Ferrannini E, Cusi K, Mandarino LJ & DeFronzo RA. (2001). Improved glycemic control and enhanced insulin sensitivity in type 2 diabetic subjects treated with pioglitazone. *Diabetes Care*, 24, 4, (Apr 2001), 710–719

Miyazaki Y, Glass L, Triplitt C, Matsuda M, Cusi K, Mahankali A, Mahankali S, Mandarino LJ & DeFronzo RA. (2001) Effect of rosiglitazone on glucose and non-esterified fatty acid metabolism in type II diabetic patients. *Diabetologia*, 44, 12, (Dec 2001), 2210–2219

Mizoguchi E, Orihara K, Hamasaki S, Ishida S, Kataoka T, Ogawa M, Saihara K, Okui H, Fukudome T, Shinsato T, Shirasawa T, Ichiki H, Kubozono T, Ninomiya Y, Otsuji Y & Tei C. (2007). Association between Toll-like receptors and the extent and severity of coronary artery disease in patients with stable angina. *Coron Artery Dis*, 18, 1, (Feb 2007), 31-38.

Monaco C, Gregan SM, Navin TJ, Foxwell BM, Davies AH & Feldmann M. (2009). Toll-like receptor-2 mediates inflammation and matrix degradation in human atherosclerosis. *Circulation*, 120, 24, (Dec 2009), 2462-2469

Moreno PR & Fuster V. (2004) New aspects in the pathogenesis of diabetic atherothrombosis. *J Am Coll Cardiol.*, 44, 12, (Dec2004),2293-2300

Morris MF. (2003). Insulin receptor signaling and regulation, In: *Textbook of Diabetes. 3rd ed.* Pickup JC, Williams G, p. 14.1–14.17, Eds. Oxford, U.K.

Müller S, Martin S, Koenig W, Hanifi-Moghaddam P, Rathmann W, Haastert B, Giani G, Illig T, Thorand B & Kolb H. (2002). Impaired glucose tolerance is associated with increased serum concentrations of interleukin 6 and co-regulated acute phase proteins but not TNF-α or its receptors. *Diabetologia*, 45, 6, (Jun 2002),805–812

Murcia AM, Hennekens CH, Lamas GA, Jiménez-Navarro M, Rouleau JL, Flaker GC, Goldman S, Skali H, Braunwald E & Pfeffer MA. (2004). Impact of diabetes on mortality in patients with myocardial infarction and left ventricular dysfunction. *Arch Intern Med*,164, 20, (Nov 2004), 2273-2279

Nakajima T, Schulte S, Warrington KJ, Kopecky SL, Frye RL, Goronzy JJ & Weyand CM. (2002). T-cell-mediated lysis of endothelial cells in acute coronary syndromes. *Circulation*, 105, 5, (Feb 2002), 570-575

Nakanishi N, Yoshida H, Matsuo Y, Suzuki K & Tatara K. (2002). White blood-cell count and the risk of impaired fasting glucose or type II diabetes in middle-aged Japanese men. *Diabetologia*, 45, 1, (Jan 2002), 42–48

Niessner A, Steiner S, Speidl WS, Pleiner J, Seidinger D, Maurer G, Goronzy JJ, Weyand CM, Kopp CW, Huber K, Wolzt M & Wojta J. (2006). Simvastatin suppresses endotoxin-induced upregulation of toll-like receptors 4 and 2 in vitro. *Atherosclerosis*, 189, 2, (Dec 2006), 408–413

Nikolajczyk BS, Jagannathan-Bogdan M, Shin H & Gyurko R. (2011). State of the union between metabolism and the immune system in type 2 diabetes. *Genes Immun*, 12, 4, (Jun 2011), 239-250

Oka S, Yoshihara E, Bizen-Abe A, Liu W, Watanabe M, Yodoi J & Masutani H. (2009). Thioredoxin binding protein-2/thioredoxin-interacting protein is a critical regulator of insulin secretion and peroxisome proliferator-activated receptor function. *Endocrinology*, 150, 3, (Mar 2009), 1225-1234

Osborn O, Brownell SE, Sanchez-Alavez M, Salomon D, Gram H & Bartfai T. (2008). Treatment with an Interleukin 1 beta antibody improves glycemic control in diet-induced obesity. *Cytokine*,44,1, (Oct 2008),141–148

Otsui K, Inoue N, Kobayashi S, Shiraki R, Honjo T, Takahashi M, Hirata K, Kawashima S & Yokoyama M. (2007). Enhanced expression of TLR4 in smooth muscle cells in human atherosclerotic coronary arteries. *Heart Vessels*, 22, 6, (Nov 2007), 416–422

Parikh H, Carlsson E, Chutkow WA, Johansson LE, Storgaard H, Poulsen P, Saxena R, Ladd C, Schulze PC, Mazzini MJ, Jensen CB, Krook A, Björnholm M, Tornqvist H, Zierath JR, Ridderstråle M, Altshuler D, Lee RT, Vaag A, Groop LC & Mootha VK. (2007). TXNIP regulates peripheral glucose metabolism in humans. *PLoS Med*, 4, 5, (May 2007) e158

Patel A, MacMahon S, Chalmers J, Neal B, Billot L, Woodward M, Marre M, Cooper M, Glasziou P, Grobbee D, Hamet P, Harrap S, Heller S, Liu L, Mancia G, Mogensen CE, Pan C, Poulter N, Rodgers A, Williams B, Bompoint S, de Galan BE, Joshi R & Travert F, ADVANCE Collaborative Group. (2008). Intensive blood-glucose control and cardiovascular outcomes in patients with type 2 diabetes. *NEJM*,358,24,(Jun 2008),2560-2572

Pickup JC, Chusney GC, Thomas SM & Burt D. (2000). Plasma interleukin-6, tumor necrosis factor alpha and blood cytokine production in types 2 diabetes. *Life Sci*, 67, 3, (Jun 2000),291–300

Pickup JC. (2003). Inflammation and activated innate immunity in the pathogenesis of type 2 diabetes. *Diabetes Care*, 27, 3, (Mar 2004), 813-823

Pitocco D, Giubilato S, Zaccardi F, Di Stasio E, Buffon A, Biasucci LM, Liuzzo G, Crea F & Ghirlanda G. (2009). Pioglitazone reduces monocyte activation in type 2 diabetes. *Acta Diabetol*, 46,1, (Mar 2009), 75-77.

Pradhan AD, Manson JE, Rifai N, Buring JE & Ridker PM. (2001). C-reactive protein, interleukin 6, and risk of developing type 2 diabetes mellitus. *JAMA*, 286, 3, (Jul 2001),327–334

Prakash MS, Chennaiah S, Murthy YS, Anjaiah E, Rao SA & Suresh C. (2006). Altered adenosine deaminase activity in type 2 diabetes mellitus. *JIACM*,7, (2006), 114-117

Rajamäki K, Lappalainen J, Oörni K, Välimäki E, Matikainen S, Kovanen PT & Eklund KK. (2010). Cholesterol crystals activate the NLRP3 inflammasome in human macrophages: a novel link between cholesterol metabolism and inflammation. *PLoSONE*, 5, 7, (Jul 2010), e11765

Randolph DA & Fathman CG. (2006). CD4+CD25+ regulatory T cells and their therapeutic potential. *Annu Rev Med*, 57, (2006), 381–402

Reimers JI. (1998). Interleukin-1 beta induced transient diabetes mellitus in rats. A model of the initial events in the pathogenesis of insulin-dependent diabetes mellitus? *Dan. Med. Bull.*, 45, 2 (Apr 1998), 45:157–180.

Richardson AP & Tayek JA. (2002). Type 2 diabetic patients may have a mild form of an injury response: a clinical research center study. *Am J Physiol*, 282,6, (Jun 2002); 1286-1290

Rodriguez-Moran M & Guerrero-Romero F. (1999). Increased levels of C-reactive protein in noncontrolled type II diabetic subjects. *J Diabetes Complications*,13, 4, (Jul-Aug 1999),211–215

Sakkinen PA, Wahl P, Cushman M, Lewis MR & Tracey RP. (2000) Clustering of procoagulation, inflammation and fibrinolysis variables with metabolic factors in insulin resistance syndrome. *Am J Epidemiol*,152, 10, (May 2000), 897–907

Sato K, Niessner A, Kopecky SL, Frye RL, Goronzy JJ & Weyand CM. (2006). TRAIL-expressing T cells induce apoptosis of vascular smooth muscle cells in the atherosclerotic plaque. *J Experim Med*, 203, 1, (Jan 2006), 239-250

Schmidt MI, Duncan BB, Sharrett AR, Lindberg G, Savage PJ, Offenbacher S, Azambuja MI, Tracy RP & Heiss G. (1999). Markers of inflammation and prediction of diabetes mellitus in adults (Atherosclerosis Risk in Communities study): a cohort study. *Lancet*, 353, 9165, (May 1999), 1649–1652

Schramm TK, Gislason GH, Køber L, Rasmussen S, Rasmussen JN, Abildstrøm SZ, Hansen ML, Folke F, Buch P, Madsen M, Vaag A & Torp-Pedersen C. (2008). Diabetes patients requiring glucose-lowering therapy and nondiabetics with a prior myocardial infarction carry the same cardiovascular risk: a population study of 3.3 million people. *Circulation*, 117, 15, (Apr 2008), 1945–1954

Schroder K & Tschopp J. (2010). The inflammasomes. *Cell*, 140, 6, (Mar 2010), 821–832

Schwartz EA, Zhang WY, Karnik SK, Borwege S, Anand VR, Laine PS, Su Y & Reaven PD. (2010). Nutrient modification of the innate immune response: a novel mechanism by which saturated fatty acids greatly amplify monocyte inflammation. *Arterioscler Thromb Vasc Biol*, 30, 4, (Apr 2010), 802–808

Seino, S & Study Group of Comprehensive Analysis of Genetic Factors in Diabetes Mellitus. (2001). S20G mutation of the amylin gene is associated with type II diabetes in Japanese.

Study Group of Comprehensive Analysis of Genetic Factors in Diabetes Mellitus. *Diabetologia*,44, 7, (Jul 2001), 906–909

Shah C, Yang G, Lee I, Bielawski J, Hannun YA & Samad F. (2008). Protection from high fat diet-induced increase in ceramide in mice lacking plasminogen activator inhibitor 1. *J Biol Chem*, 283 ,20, (May 2008), 13538-13548

Shindler DM, Palmeri ST, Antonelli TA, Sleeper LA, Boland J, Cocke TP & Hochman JS. (2000). Diabetes mellitus in cardiogenic shock complicated acute myocardial infarction: a report from the SHOCK trial registry. Should we emergently revascularize occluded coronaries for cardiogenic shock? *J Am Coll Cardiol*, 36, 3 (Suppl A), (Sep 2000), 1097-1103.

Shinohara M, Hirata K, Yamashita T, Takaya T, Sasaki N, Shiraki R, Ueyama T, Emoto N, Inoue N, Yokoyama M & Kawashima S.(2007). Local overexpression of toll-like receptors at the vessel wall induces atherosclerotic lesion formation: synergism of TLR2 and TLR4. *Arterioscler Thromb Vasc Biol*, 27, 11, (Nov 2007), 2384-2391

Shiraki R, Inoue N, Kobayashi S, Ejiri J, Otsui K, Honjo T, Takahashi M, Hirata K, Yokoyama M & Kawashima S. (2006). Toll-like receptor 4 expressions on peripheral blood monocytes were enhanced in coronary artery disease even in patients with low C-reactive protein. *Life Sci*, 80, 1, (Dec 2006), 59-66

Snijder MB, Dekker JM, Visser M, Stehouwer CDA, van Hinsberg VWM, Bouter LM & Heine RJ. (2001). C-reactive protein and diabetes mellitus type 2. *Diabetologia*, 44, (2001), 115

Spranger J, Kroke A, Möhlig M, Hoffmann K, Bergmann MM, Ristow M, Boeing H & Pfeiffer AF. (2003). Inflammatory cytokines and the risk to develop type 2 diabetes: results of the prospective population-based European Prospective Investigation into Cancer and Nutrition (EPIC)-Potsdam study. *Diabetes*, 52, 3, (Mar 2003), 812–817

Sriharan M, Reichelt AJ, Opperman ML, Duncan BB, Mengue SS, Crook MA & Schmidt MI. (2002). Total sialic acid and associated elements of the metabolic syndrome in women with and without previous gestational diabetes. *Diabetes Care*,25, 8, (Aug 2002), 1331–1335

Stienstra R, Joosten LA, Koenen T, van Tits B, van Diepen JA, van den Berg SA, Rensen PC, Voshol PJ, Fantuzzi G, Hijmans A, Kersten S, Müller M, van den Berg WB, van Rooijen N, Wabitsch M, Kullberg BJ, van der Meer JW, Kanneganti T, Tack CJ, & Netea MG. (2010). The inflammasome-mediated caspase-1 activation controls adipocyte differentiation and insulin sensitivity. *Cell Metab*, 12, 6, (Dec 2010), 593-605

Stienstra R, van Diepen JA, Tack CJ, Zaki MH, van de Veerdonk FL, Perera D, Neale GA, Hooiveld GJ, Hijmans A, Vroegrijk I, van den Berg S, Romijn J, Rensen PC, Joosten LA, Netea MG & Kanneganti TD.(2011). Inflammasome is a central player in the induction of obesity and insulin resistance. *Proc Natl Acad Sci*, 108, 37, (Sep 2011), 15324-15329

Stoll LL, Denning GM & Weintraub NL.(2006). Endotoxin, TLR4 signaling and vascular inflammation: potential therapeutic targets in cardiovascular disease. *Curr Pharm Des*, 12, 32, (2006),4229–4245

Strowig T, Henao-Mejia J, Elinav E & Flavell R. (2012). Inflammasomes in health and disease. *Nature*, 481, 7381, (Jan 2012),278-286

Summerfield JA, Sumiya M, Levin M & Turner MW. (1997). Association of mutations in mannose binding protein gene with childhood infection in consecutive hospital series. *BMJ*, 314, 7089, (Apr 1997),1229-32

Takeda K & Akira S. (2004). TLR signaling pathways. *Semin Immunol*, 16, 1, (Feb 2004), 3-9

Tanaka T, Itoh H, Doi K, Fukunaga Y, Hosoda K, Shintani M, Yamashita J, Chun TH, Inoue M, Masatsugu K, Sawada N, Saito T, Inoue G, Nishimura H,Yoshimasa Y & Nakao K.(1999). Down regulation of peroxisome proliferator-activated receptor-γ expression by inflammatory cytokines and its reversal by thiazolidinediones. *Diabetologia*, 42, 6, (Jun 1999),702–710

Temelkova-Kurktschiev T, Henkel E, Koehler C, Karrei K & Hanefield M. (2002). Subclinical inflammation in newly detected type II diabetes and impaired glucose tolerance. *Diabetologia*, 45, 1, (Jan 2002), 151

Temelkova-Kurktschiev T, Siegert G, Bergmann S, Henkel E, Koehler C, Jaross W & Hanefeld M. (2002). Subclinical inflammation is strongly related to insulin resistance but not insulin secretion in a high risk population for diabetes. *Metabolism*, 51, 6, (Jun 2002),743–749

Thorand B, Löwel H, Schneider A, Kolb H, Meisinger C, Fröhlich M & Koenig W. (2003). C-reactive protein as a predictor for incident diabetes mellitus among middle-aged men: results from the MONICA Augsburg cohort study. *Arch Intern Med*, 163, 1, (Jan 2003), 93–99

Tsukumo DM, Carvalho-Filho MA, Carvalheira JB, Prada PO, Hirabara SM, Schenka AA, Araújo EP, Vassallo J, Curi R, Velloso LA & Saad MJ. (2007). Loss-of-function mutation in Toll-like receptor 4 prevents diet-induced obesity and insulin resistance. *Diabetes*, 56, 8, (Aug 2007), 1986-1998

UKPDS Group. (1998). Effect of intensive blood-glucose control with metformin on complications in overweight patients with type 2 diabetes (UKPDS 34). *Lancet*, 352, 9131, (Sep 1998), 854-865

Vandanmagsar B, Youm YH, Ravussin A, Galgani JE, Stadler K, Mynatt RL, Ravussin E, Stephens JM & Dixit VD. (2011). The NLRP3 inflammasome instigates obesity-induced inflammation and insulin resistance. *Nature Med*, 17, 2, (Feb 2011), 179–188

Versteeg D, Hoefer IE, Schoneveld AH, de Kleijn DP, Busser E, Strijder C, Emons M, Stella PR, Doevendans PA & Pasterkamp G. (2008). Monocyte toll-like receptor 2 and 4 responses and expression following percutaneous coronary intervention: association with lesion stenosis and fractional flow reserve. *Heart*, 94, 6, (Jun 2008), 770-776

Visser M, Bouter LM, McQuillan GM, Wener MH & Harris TB. (1999). Elevated C-reactive protein levels in overweight and obese adults. *JAMA*, 282, 22, (Dec 1999), 2131–2135

Vozarova B, Weyer C, Lindsay RS, Pratley RE, Bogardus C & Tataranni PA. (2002). High white blood cell count is associated with a worsening of insulin sensitivity and predicts the development of type 2 diabetes. *Diabetes*,51, 2, (Feb 2002), 455–461

Wen H, Gris D, Lei Y, Jha S, Zhang L, Huang MT, Brickey WJ & Ting JP. (2011). Fatty acid-induced NLRP3-ASC inflammasome activation interferes with insulin signaling. *Nat Immunol*, 12, 5, (May 2011), 408-415.

Weyer C, Yudkin JS, Stehouwer CD, Schalkwijk CG, Pratley RE & Tataranni PA. (2002). Humoral markers of inflammation and endothelial dysfunction in relation to adiposity and in vivo insulin action in Pima Indians. *Atherosclerosis,*161, 1, (Mar 2002), 233– 242

Wild S, Roglic G, Green A, Sicree R & King H. (2004). Global prevalence of diabetes: Estimates for the year 2000 and projections for 2030. *Diabetes Care,* 27, 5, (May 2004), 1047

Winer S, Chan Y, Paltser G, Truong D, Tsui H, Bahrami J, Dorfman R, Wang Y, Zielenski J, Mastronardi F, Maezawa Y, Drucker DJ, Engleman E, Winer D & Dosch HM. (2009). Normalization of obesity-associated insulin resistance through immunotherapy. *Nat. Med.,* 15, 8, (Aug 2009), 921–929.

Winer S, Paltser G, Chan Y, Tsui H, Engleman E, Winer D & Dosch HM. (2009). Obesity predisposes to Th17 bias. *Eur. J. Immunol.,* 39, 9, (Sep 2009), 2629–2635

Winkler G, Salamon F, Salamon D, Speer G, Simon K & Cseh K. (1998). Elevated tumor necrosis factor alpha levels can contribute to the insulin resistance in type II (non-insulin-dependent) diabetes and obesity. *Diabetologia,* 41, 7, (Jul 1998), 860–862

Wyss CA, Neidhart M, Altwegg L, Spanaus KS, Yonekawa K, Wischnewsky MB, Corti R, Kucher N, Roffi M, Eberli FR, Amann-Vesti B, Gay S, von Eckardstein A,Lüscher TF & Maier W. (2010).Cellular actors, Toll-like receptors, and local cytokine profile in acute coronary syndromes. *Eur Heart J,* 31, 12, (Jun 2010), 1457–1469

Xu XH, Shah PK, Faure E, Equils O, Thomas L, Fishbein MC, Luthringer D, Xu XP, Rajavashisth TB, Yano J, Kaul S & Arditi M. (2001). Toll-like receptor-4 is expressed by macrophages in murine and human lipid-rich atherosclerotic plaques and upregulated by oxidized LDL. *Circulation,* 104, 25, (Dec 2001), 3103–3108

Yang L, Anderson DE, Baecher-Allan C, Hastings WD, Bettelli E, Oukka M, Kuchroo VK & Hafler DA. (2008). IL-21 and TGF-beta are required for differentiation of human Th17 cells. *Nature,* 454, 7202, (Jul 2008) 350–352

Yonekawa K, Neidhart M, Altwegg LA, Wyss CA, Corti R, Vogl T, Grigorian M, Gay S, Lüscher TF & Maier W. (2011). Myeloid related proteins activate Toll-like receptor 4 in human acute coronary syndromes. *Atherosclerosis,* 218, 2, (Oct 2011), 486-92.

Yudkin JS, Stehouwer CD, Emeis JJ & Coppack SW. (1999). C-reactive protein in healthy subjects: association with obesity, insulin resistance, and endothelial dysfunction: a potential role for cytokines originating from the adipose tissue? *Arterioscler Thromb Vasc Biol* , 19, 4, (Apr 1999), 972–978

Zhou R, Tardivel A, Thorens B, Choi I & Tschopp J. (2010). Thioredoxin-interacting protein links oxidative stress to inflammasome activation. *Nature Immunol,* 11, 2, (Feb 2010) 136–140.

Chapter 4

Diabetic Nephropathy

Božidar Vujičić, Tamara Turk, Željka Crnčević-Orlić,
Gordana Đorđević and Sanjin Rački

Additional information is available at the end of the chapter

http://dx.doi.org/10.5772/50115

1. Introduction

Diabetes mellitus (DM) is the most frequent cause of chronic kidney failure in both developed and developing countries [1]. Diabetic nephropathy, also known as Kimmelstiel-Wilson syndrome or nodular diabetic glomerulosclerosis or intercapillary glomerulonephritis, is a clinical syndrome characterized by albuminuria (>300 mg/day or >200 mcg/min) confirmed on at least two occasions 3-6 months apart, permanent and irreversible decrease in glomerular filtration rate (GFR) (Table 1), and arterial hypertension [2]. The syndrome was first described by a British physician Clifford Wilson (1906-1997) and American physician Paul Kimmelstiel (1900-1970) in 1936 [3].

	Decline in glomerular filtration rate (ml/min/year)	
Diabetes	Type 1	Type 2
Normoalbuminuria	1,2 - 3,6	0,96
Microalbuminuria	1,2 - 3,6	2,4
Proteinuria	9,6 - 12	5,4 - 7,2

Table 1. Decline in glomerular filtration rate in various stages of type 1 and type 2 diabetes. Available: http://emedicine.medscape.com/article/238946-overview. Accessed 2012 May 14

Diabetic nephropathy is a chronic complication of both type 1 DM (beta cell destruction – absolute lack of insulin) and type 2 DM (insulin resistance and/or decreased secretion of insulin) [4]. There are five stages in the development of diabetic nephropathy.

Stage I: Hypertrophic hyper filtration. In this stage, GFR is either normal or increased. Stage I lasts approximately five years from the onset of the disease. The size of the kidneys is increased by approximately 20% and renal plasma flow is increased by 10%-15%, while albuminuria and blood pressure remain within the normal range.

Stage II: The quiet stage. This stage starts approximately two years after the onset of the disease and is characterized by kidney damage with basement membrane thickening and mesangial proliferation. There are still no clinical signs of the disease. GFR returns to normal values. Many patients remain in this stage until the end of their life.

Stage III: The microalbuminuria stage (albumin 30-300 mg/dU) or initial nephropathy. This is the first clinically detectable sign of glomerular damage. It usually occurs five to ten years after the onset of the disease. Blood pressure may be increased or normal. Approximately 40% of patients reach this stage.

Stage IV: Chronic kidney failure (CKF) is the irreversible stage. Proteinuria develops (albumin > 300 mg/dU), GFR decreases below 60 mL/min/1.73 m^2, and blood pressure increases above normal values.

Stage V: Terminal kidney failure (TKF) (GFR < 15 mL/min/1.73 m^2). Approximately 50% of the patients with TKF require kidney replacement therapy (peritoneal dialysis, hemodialysis, kidney transplantation) [5].

In the initial stages of diabetic nephropathy, increased kidney size and changed Doppler indicators may be the early morphological signs of renal damage, while proteinuria and GFR are the best indicators of the degree of the damage [6].

2. Epidemiology

The prognostic value of a small amount of albumin in urine for the development of kidney damage in patients with type 1 or 2 DM was confirmed in the early 1980's. This stage of kidney damage was called the microalbuminuria stage or initial nephropathy [7]. Approximately 20-30% of the patients develop microalbuminuria after 15 years of disease duration and less than half develop real nephropathy [8]. The European Diabetes (EURODIAB) Prospective Complications Study Group [9] and 18-year Danish study [10] showed that the overall occurrence of microalbuminuria in patients with type 1 and 2 DM is 12.6% (after 7.3 years) and 33%, respectively. According to the United Kingdom Prospective Diabetes Study (UKPDS), the annual incidence of microalbuminuria in patients with type 2 DM in Great Britain is 2% and the prevalence is 25% ten years after the diagnosis [2]. Proteinuria develops in approximately 15-40% patients with type 1 DM, usually after 15-20 years of DM duration [11]. In patients with type 2 DM, the prevalence varies between 5% and 20% on average [2]. Diabetic nephropathy is more frequent in African Americans, Asian Americans, and Native Americans [12]. In Caucasians, the progressive kidney disease is more frequent in patients with type 1 than type 2 DM, although its overall prevalence in the diabetic population is higher in patients with type 2 DM because this type of DM is more prevalent [13]. The occurrence of diabetic nephropathy in Pima Indians is very interesting, indeed. According to a study published in 1990, around 50% of Pima Indians with type 2 DM developed nephropathy after 20 years of the disease, and 15% of them were already in the terminal stage of kidney failure [14].

In the United States, the occurrence of diabetic nephropathy in patients beginning kidney replacement therapy doubled in the 1991-2001 period [12]. Fortunately, the trend has been decreasing, most likely due to the better prevention and earlier diagnosis and treatment of DM [15].

3. Pathology

Glomerular filtration barrier functions as a complex biological sieve. As opposed to other capillaries in the body, glomerular capillaries are highly permeable to water (hydraulic conductivity) and relatively impermeable to large molecules. Such permeability is possible because of the unique three-layer structure of glomerular filtration membrane consisting of endothelial glycocalyx, glomerular basement membrane, and podocytes (glomerular visceral epithelial cells). Pathological changes develop in the glomeruli of patients with long-duration DM before the appearance of microalbuminuria.

The severity of glomerular damage is proportional to GFR value, DM duration, and blood glucose regulation [16,17]. The main pathohystological changes in diabetic nephropathy include the thickening of the glomerular basement membrane (GBM), mesangial expansion, nodular sclerosis – Kimmelstiel-Wilson change, diffuse glomerular sclerosis, tubular interstitial fibrosis, and arteriosclerosis and hyalinosis of kidney blood vessels (Figures 1-3).

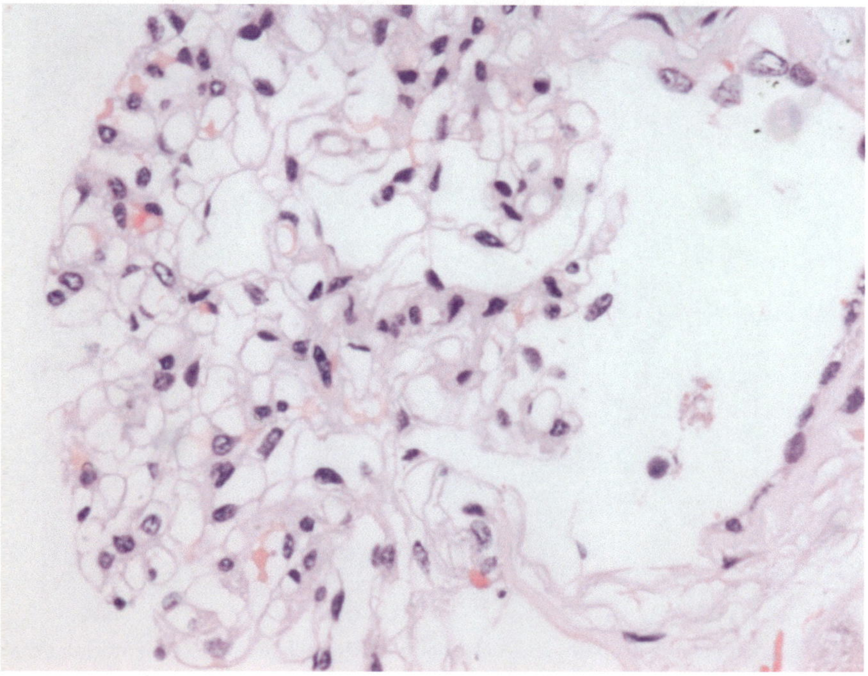

Figure 1. Photography shows delicate structure of normal glomerulus with thin glomerular basement membrane and unrecognizable mesangium. HE stain, X 400.

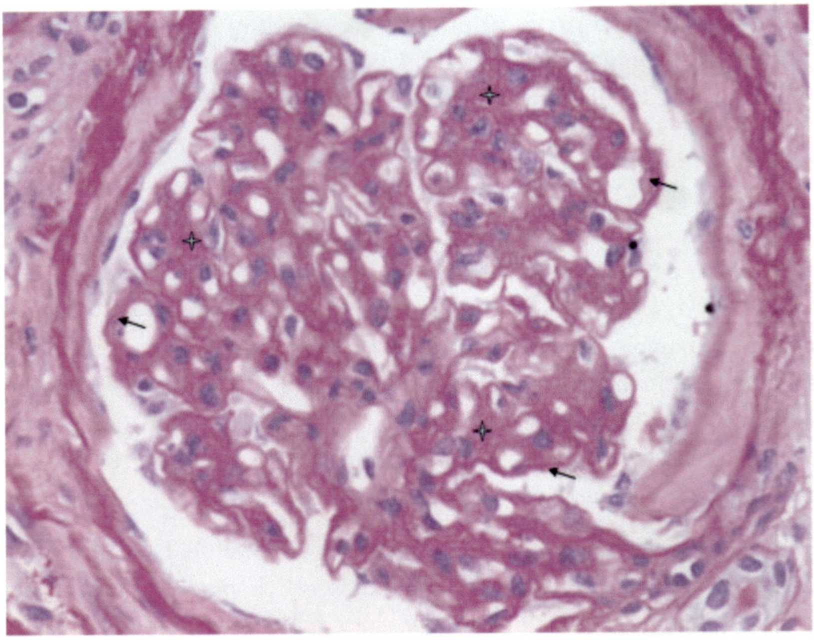

Figure 2. Class II b diabetic nephropathy. Diffuse expansion of mesangium (star) and diffuse thickening of the glomerular basement membrane (arrow). PAS stain, X400.

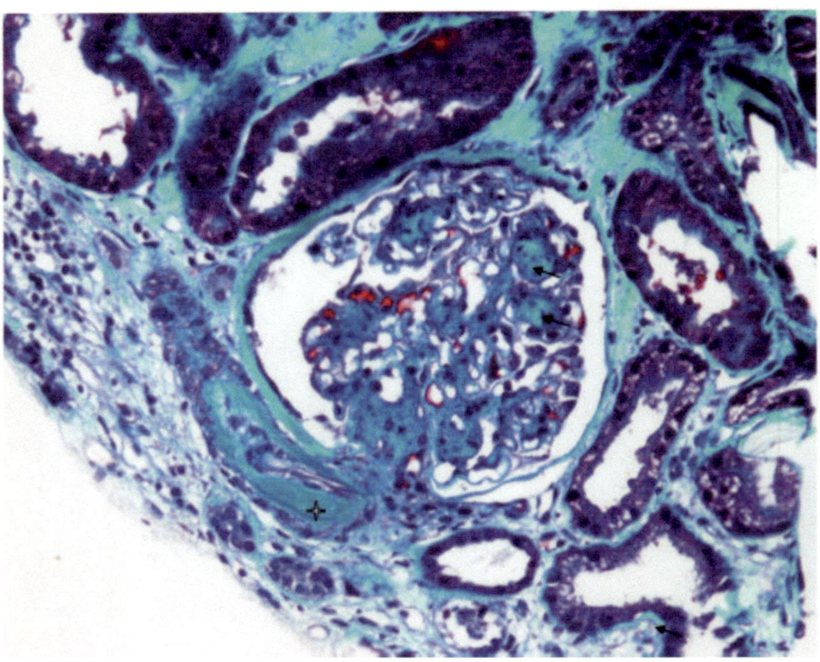

Figure 3. Class III diabetic nephropathy. Sclerotic nodule (Kimmelstiel–Wilson) in nodular diabetic nephropathy (arrow). Afferent and efferent arteriolar hyalinosis is characteristic for diabetic nephropathy (star). The arrow in the lower right corner indicates thickening of the tubular basement membrane. Mallory stain, X 100.

Among other pathological lesions, we should mention hyalinosis, the so-called fibrin cap, which consists of accumulated hyaline material between endothelial cells and glomerular basement membrane (Figure 4) [18]. Fibrin cap is present in approximately 60% of the cases and is believed to be associated with chronic ischemia [19].

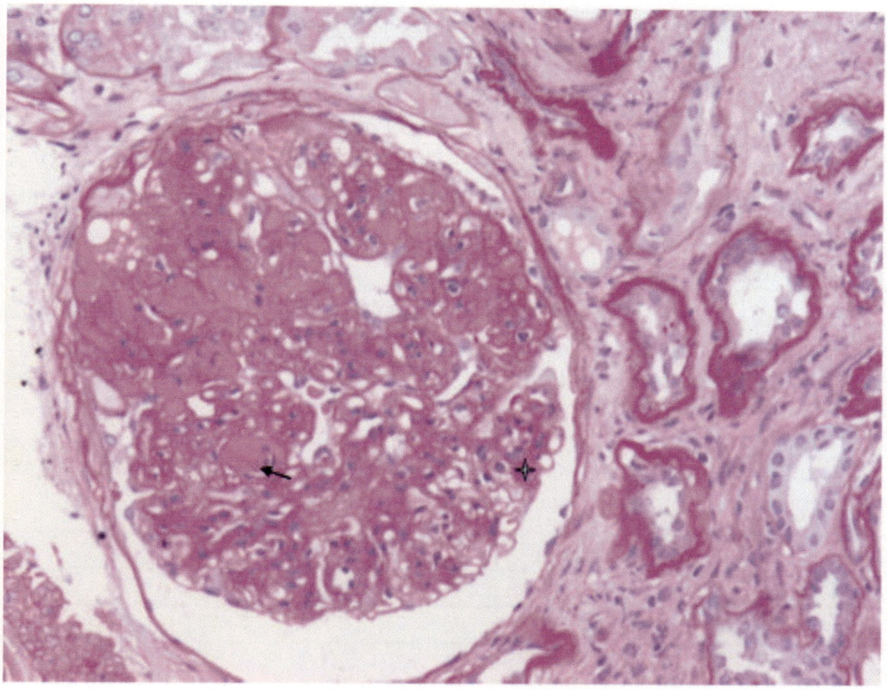

Figure 4. Fibrin cap (arrow) is characteristic for diabetic nephropathy. It is caused by insudation and accumulation of glycosilated plasma proteins between the glomerular endothelium and the glomerular basement membrane. Diffuse expansion of mesangium is designated by four point star. PAS stain, X 200.

There is a significant overlap between the described changes in patients in different stages of albuminuria, independent of their type of DM [16]. All histological patterns have identical prognostic significance (Figures 5,6). However, the fact that the expansion of mesangium and glomerular sclerosis do not occur simultaneously indicates their different pathogenesis within diabetic nephropathy [20]. Under light microscopy, the reduction in the podocyte number is easily noticed in patients with type 1 DM and 2 [21].

Since histological changes in both types of DM overlap to a great extent, the Scientific Committee of the Society for Pathological Anatomy established the Pathologic Classification of Diabetic Nephropathy, where diabetic nephropathy is histologically divided into four stages of glomerular damage (Table 2).

Class	Description	Inclusion criteria
I	Mild or nonspecific LM changes and EM-proven GBM thickening	Biopsy does not meet any of the criteria mentioned below for class II, III, or IV GBM 395 nm in female and 430 nm in male individuals 9 years of age and older[a]
II a	Mild mesangial expansion	Biopsy does not meet criteria for class III or IV Mild mesangial expansion in 25% of the observed mesangium
II b	Severe mesangial expansion	Biopsy does not meet criteria for class III or IV Severe mesangial expansion in 25% of the observed mesangium
III	Nodular sclerosis (Kimmelstiel – Wilson lesion)	Biopsy does not meet criteria for class IV At least one convincing Kimmelstiel –Wilson lesion
IV	Advanced diabetic glomerulosclerosis	Global glomerular sclerosis in 50% of Glomeruli Lesions from classes I through III

Table 2. Four classes of glomerular lesions in diabetic nephropathy. Adapted from [22].
LM, light microscopy. EM, electronic microscopy. GBM, glomerular basement membrane.
[a] On the basis of direct measurement of GBM width by EM, these individual cutoff levels may be considered indicative when other GBM measurements are used.

The same group of international experts established the histological scoring system for the changes in the interstitium and relevant blood vessels (Table 3) [22].

Lesion	Criteria	Score
Interstitial lesions		
IFTA	No IFTA	0
	< 25%	1
	25% - 50%	2
	> 50%	3
interstitial inflammation	Absent	0
	Infiltration only in relation to IFTA	1
	Infiltration in areas without IFTA	2
Vascular lesions		
arteriolar hyalinosis	Absent	0
	At least one area of arteriolar hyalinosis	1
	More than one area of arteriolar hyalinosis	2
presence of large vessels		Yes/No
arteriosclerosis (score worst artery)	No intimal thickening	0
	Intimal thickening less than thickness of media	1
	Intimal thickening greater than thickness of media	2

Table 3. Interstitial and vascular lesions of diabetic nephropaty. Adapted from [22].
IFTA, interstitial fibrosis and tubular athrophy.

In addition to diabetic nephropathy, glomerular sclerosis can also develop in other pathological conditions in patients with DM. These are:

a. dysproteinemia (amyloidosis and other deposit diseases)
b. conditions with chronic ischemia (cyanotic congenital heart disease)
c. chronic membranoproliferative glomerulonephritis
d. Idiopathic diseases mostly associated with smoking and increased blood pressure [23].

It means that pathological findings in the urine of patients with DM (proteinuria and erythrocyturia) are not necessarily the result of diabetic nephropathy and should not be considered as such. This finding is a diagnostic challenge for a clinician as well as pathologist [24]. Therefore, in case of hematuria, more severe nephrotic syndrome, and/or rapidly advancing deterioration of renal function without concomitant diabetic nephropathy in patients with DM, we should consider an underlying non-diabetic kidney disease. Kidney biopsy with a complete analysis of the sample (light, immunofluorescent, and electron microscopies) represents the gold standard in the diagnostic workup of patients with non-diabetic renal disease. Always correlate the biopsy findings with the clinical history. If the patient is not diabetic, consider the diagnosis of idiopathic nodular glomerulosclerosis

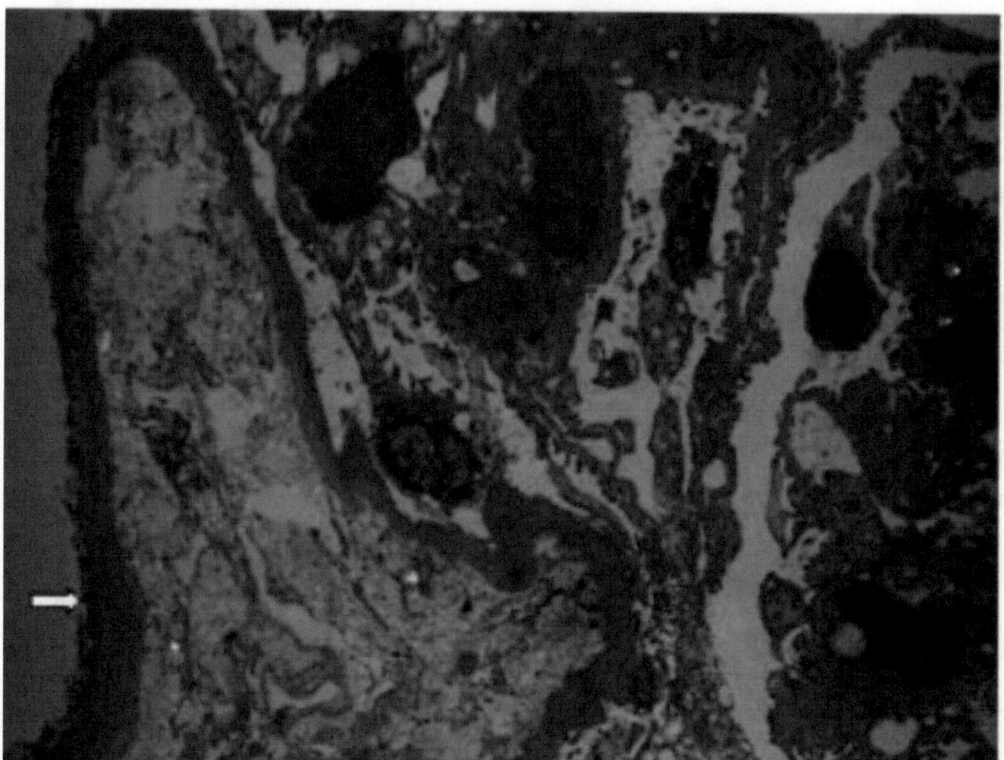

Figure 5. There was marked thickening, irregularity of the basement membrane of the capillary wall with lamellation (electron microscopy, arrow, 2.8 k)

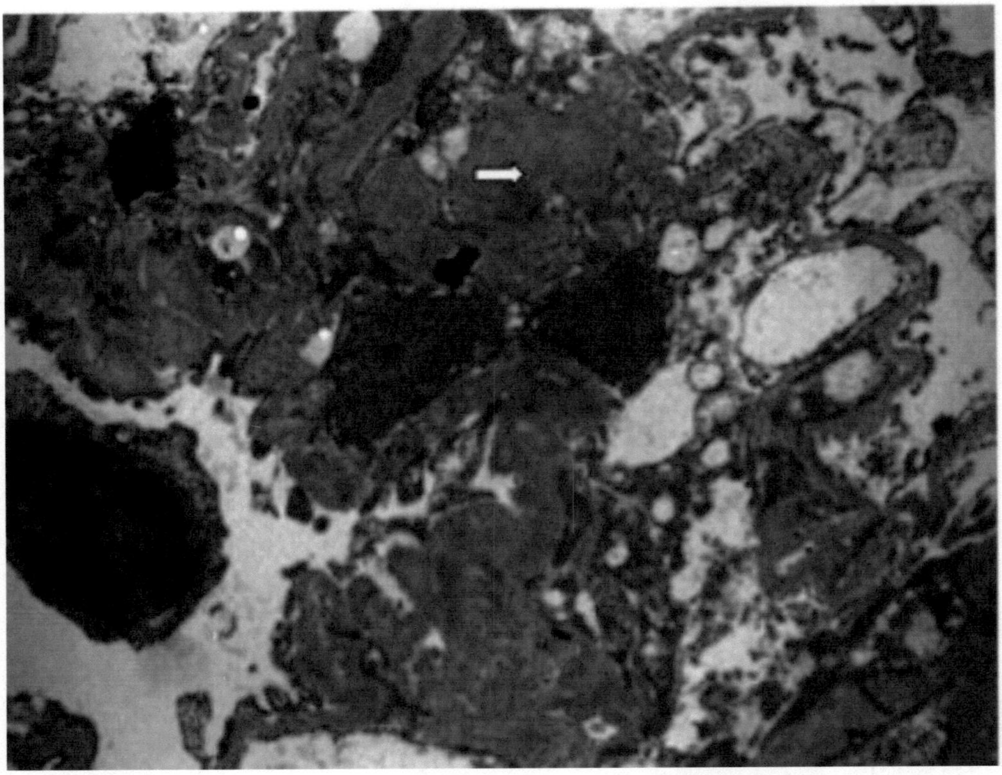

Figure 6. Mesangial regions are also expanded by excess mesangial matrix-like material (electron microscopy, arrow, 7.1 k)

If primary glomerular disease is found in a patient with DM, with or without diabetic nephropathy, the therapeutic approach changes as well as the course and outcome of the renal disease [25].

4. Pathogenesis

Pathogenesis of diabetic nephropathy is very complicated and results from the interaction of hemodynamic and metabolic factors.

Glomerular hyper filtration

Increased intraglomerular pressure and hyper filtration as early changes in the development of diabetic nephropathy were described by Stadler and Schmidt in 1959 [26]. In the 1970's, Mogensen emphasized that as many as 40% newly found DM cases had increased glomerular filtration [27].

Although the mechanism of development of hyper filtration is not completely understood, several factors have been found to play a role in its development.

Hormones

The role of hormones was experimentally demonstrated in the study by Serri et al, who showed that the infusion of somatostatin analogues (octreotide) partly led to the decrease in hyperfiltration and kidney size. In their study, glycemic regulation, plasma glucagon, and growth hormone levels remained unchanged, but the concentration of insulin-like growth factor-1 (IGF-1) decreased [28]. Pathogenetic role of IGF-1 has not been completely elucidated, but it is known that exogenous administration of his hormone in non-DM patients leads to afferent arteriolar dilation and GFR increase, which are the changes also observed in initial diabetic nephropathy [29]. The identical hemodynamic changes, along with the increase in kidney size, occur in experimental animal models after the infusion of IGF-1 [30]. Sex hormones may also influence hyperfiltration. Cherney et al. [31] observed a decrease in kidney blood flow and vascular resistance in response to hyperglycemia in women, but not in men. The same study showed that the addition of angiotensin-converting enzyme inhibitor (ACEI) resulted in a decrease in blood pressure in both men and women, but GFR decreased only in women [31].

Sorbitol

The enzyme aldose reductase converts intracellular glucose to sorbitol, which remains in the cell. Although research in patients with type 1 DM and known hyperfiltration has shown that the infusion of aldose reductase inhibitor (tolrestat) decreases GFR to normal values, a possible therapeutic use of this agent should be confirmed in more studies [32].

Increased sodium reabsorption and tubuloglomerular feedback

Increased renal tubular sodium reabsorption due to increased sodium-glucose co-transport leads to the increase in extracellular fluid volume, which then increases GFR [33]. In an experimental DM model, it was shown that hyperinsulinemia and mild hyperglycemia stimulate reabsorption of sodium in the proximal tubules, resulting in the decreased fluid flow to distal tubules, which then activates the so-called tubuloglomerular feedback mechanism in the macula densa [34]. This causes the afferent arteriole dilation and leads to an increase in the GFR. In this case, the renal hyper filtration response to the imbalance caused by increased sodium reabsorption in the proximal tubules consequently increases fluid retention. Although the role of glomerular hyperfiltration in the pathogenesis of diabetic nephropathy is unquestionable, it itself is not sufficient to cause kidney damage.

Poor control of metabolic factors

Glycation end-products

Part of the excess glucose in chronic hyperglycemia binds to free amino acids of circulating or tissue proteins. This non-enzymatic process produces reversible early glycation products, and later, irreversible advanced glycation end products (AGEs), which accumulate in the tissues and contribute to the development of microvascular complications of DM [35].

AGEs modulate the cell activation, signal transduction, and cytokine and growth factor expression through the activation of R-dependent and R-independent signal pathways. Bonding to their podocyte receptors, AGEs may induce expression of some factors considered to play the key role in the pathogenesis of diabetic nephropathy, such as transforming growth factor-beta (TGF-beta) and connective tissue growth factor (CTGF) [36]. In non-diabetic mice, the infusion of early products of glycation up to the concentration seen in diabetic mice increases the kidneys blood flow, GFR, and intraglomerular pressure, which are characteristic of untreated DM [37].

Hyperglycemia

The evidence from *in vitro* studies shows that hyperglycemia has a direct effect on mesangial cell proliferation, matrix expansion, and glycosylation of glomerular proteins [38,39].

Protein kinase C

The activation of protein kinase C (PKC) is one of the main mediators of hyperglycemia-induced tissue injury. PCK activation leads to increased vascular permeability, increased synthesis of extracellular matrix components, and increased production of reactive oxygen species (ROS), which are important mediators of kidney injury [40].

Heparanase Expression

The regulation of heparanase expression plays an important role in the pathogenesis of diabetic nephropathy. The reduction in heparin sulfate on the surface of endothelial cell changes the negative charge of glycocalyx and consequently increases albumin permeability of the glomerular filtration membrane [41].

Reactive Oxygen Species

Increasing evidence shows the importance of reactive oxygen species (ROS) in the pathogenesis of diabetic nephropathy. Although the ROS production may be influenced by numerous mechanisms, the most important role in their production is played by superoxide produced by glycolysis and oxidative phosphorylation in the mitochondria. ROS activate all important pathogenetic mechanisms, such as increased production of AGEs, increased glucose entry into the polyol pathway, and PKC activation [42]. In addition, ROS directly damage endothelial glycocalyx, which leads to albuminuria without the concurrent damage to the GBM itself.

Prorenin

Increased serum prorenin plays a role in the development of diabetic nephropathy in children and adolescents [43]. Prorenin binds to a specific tissue receptor, leading to the activation of the signal pathway of mitogen-activating protein kinases (MAPK), which potentiate the development of kidney damage [44]. Using an experimental model of diabetic nephropathy, Ichihara et al. [45] indicated a possible role of prorenin in the development of diabetic nephropathy. In their study, a prolonged prorenin receptor blockade cancelled the activation of MAPK, which prevented the development of diabetic nephropathy despite the increased activity of angiotensine II.

Cytokines and Growth Factors

Hyperglycemia stimulates increased expression of different growth factors and activation of cytokines, which overall contributes to further kidney damage [46,47].

In the kidney biopsy samples from patients with type 2 DM, a significant increase in platelet derived growth factor (PDGF) expression was found. Moreover, the site of expression of this factor is adjacent to the areas of interstitial fibrosis, which is important in the pathogenesis of fibrosis in kidney injury [48].

Hyperglycemia also increases the glomerular expression of TGF-beta; matrix proteins are specifically stimulated by this growth factor [49]. Furthermore, the expression of bone morphogenic protein 7 (BMP-7) in DM is decreased, and the expression of profibrinogenic TGF-beta is increased [50,51].

Nephrine Expression

Nephrine is a transmembrane protein, the main structural element in *slit* diaphragm and as such, it is important for the maintenance of filtration membrane integrity. More recent studies have shown the association between the decreased expression of nephrine and albuminuria progression in the model of human diabetic nephropathy [52,53].

5. Risk factors

There are several risk factors for the development of diabetic nephropathy. They can be divided into those that cannot be altered (genetic factors, age, and race) and those that can and must be changed (hyperglycemia, hypertension, dyslipidemia, and GFR) [53].

Genetic Predisposition

Genetic predisposition substantially determines the occurrence and severity of diabetic nephropathy [18,40]. The likeliness of diabetic nephropathy is higher in siblings and children of parents with diabetic nephropathy, independently of the type of DM [54]. There is a 14% probability for a child of the parents without proteinuria to develop clinical proteinuria, 23% probabilities in cases where one of the parents has proteinuria, and 46% probability in case that both parents have proteinuria. This increased risk cannot be explained by the duration of DM, increased blood pressure or gycemic regulation. However, genetic predisposition for excessive salt intake and arterial hypertension could play a role. Although likeliness of chromosomes 3, 7, 18, and 20 to be associated with diabetic nephropathy is relatively high, we still cannot confirm the role of particular predisposing genetic determinants due to inconsistent results of the studies of genetic factors important in the development of this disease.

Race

The incidence of diabetic nephropathy is increased in African American, Mexican American, and Asian Indian ethnic groups. Occurrence and severity of the disease are higher in Blacks

(3- to 6-fold in comparison with Caucasians), American Mexicans, and especially in Pima Indians in the North West part of the United States [55]. This observation in genetically incongruent populations suggests that socioeconomic factors, such as nutrition and poor control of glycemia, blood pressure, and body weight, play the key role.

Age

In patients with type 2 DM, age and duration of DM increase the risk for albuminuria [53]. In the population study of 1586 Pima Indians with type 2 DM, subjects diagnosed with DM before age 20 had a higher risk of developing terminal kidney failure (25 vs. 5 patients in 1000 incident patients). According to Svensson et al. [56] the risk of terminal kidney failure in patients with type 1 DM was low if the disease was diagnosed by the age of 5.

Increased Blood Pressure

There is a high prevalence rate of hypertension in patients with type 1 DM (40%) and type 2 DM (70%), even before albuminuria can be found.

Evidence from several large clinical studies (UKPDS, ADVANCE) indicates a causal relationship between the increased arterial pressure and diabetic nephropathy [57]. Moreover, at least three factors have been shown to contribute to the development of increased arterial pressure in this metabolic disorder including hyperinsulinemia, excessive extracellular fluid volume, and increased arterial rigidity. Hyperinsulinemia contributes to the development of increased arterial pressure via insulin resistance in type 2 DM or via administration of insulin per *se*. Randeree et al. study in 80 patients with type 2 DM who started treatment with exogenous insulin showed an increase in their blood pressure from 132/81 mm Hg to 149/89 mm Hg [58]. This hypertensive response, although not reported in all clinical studies, is most likely mediated by weight gain combined with pro-hypertensive effect of insulin. Hyperinsulinemia could be the link between overweight and increased blood pressure in patients with or without DM, since it increases sympathetic activity and retention of sodium in the kidneys.

Sodium and water retention are induced by insulin itself, while the increased filtration of glucose is induced by hyperglycemia. The excess filtered glucose is reabsorbed (as long as there is a moderate hyperglycemia) in the proximal tubule via sodium-glucose co-transport, which concurrently leads to the increase in sodium reabsorption [59]. Sodium reabsorption increases blood pressure, which may be prevented and regulated by salt-free diet.

Patients with DM have increased arterial stiffness, which develops due to the increased glycation of proteins and consequent development of arteriosclerosis. Decreased arterial elasticity in patients with glucose intolerance or DM contributes to the increased systolic pressure as an independent mortality risk factor [60].

Glomerular Filtration Rate

Increased GFR at diagnosis is a risk factor for the development of diabetic nephropathy. In approximately half of the patients with type 1 DM lasting up to five years, GFR value is approximately 25-50% above normal range. These patients have a higher risk of developing diabetic nephropathy [61].

Dynamics of structural and hemodynamic changes is influenced by increased intraglomerular pressure, with the resulting glomerular hyperfiltration and hypertrophy and damage to the endothelial wall. Strict glycemic control, limited protein intake, and blood pressure control may slow down the progress of renal disease in type 1 DM [62]. The situation with type 2 DM is somewhat different. More than 45% of patients with type 2 DM at diagnosis have GFR that is two standard deviations higher than that in their age-matched no-DM or overweight controls [63]. Granted, the hyper filtration rate (117-133 mL/min on average) is lower than that in type 1 DM. Patients with type 2 DM are older and, therefore, have greater likelihood of developing atherosclerotic vascular changes that influence GFR and glomerular size [64]. The role of intraglomerular hypertension in the pathogenesis of diabetic nephropathy explains why systemic hypertension is such an important risk factor for the development of this kidney disease [65]. Studies on animal models showed that DM is associated with damage of renal autoregulation. As a result, increased blood pressure does not induce the expected vasoconstriction in the afferent arteriole, which would reduce the influence of systemic hypertension on intraglomerular pressure [66].

Glycemic Regulation

Diabetic nephropathy often develops in patients with poor glycemic control. The degree of glycemic control is an important predictor of terminal kidney failure [67]. In Krolewski et al's [68] study, the prevalence of terminal kidney failure was 36% in patients with the worst glycemic control in comparison with 9% in the group with well-controlled glycaemia.

It is generally accepted that the degree of glycemic control is a very important risk factor for the development diabetic nephropathy.

Overweight

High body mass index (BMI) increases the risk of development of chronic kidney disease in patients with DM [53]. Furthermore, adequate diet and reduction in body weight decrease proteinuria and improve kidney function in these patients [69]. The role of overweight as a risk factor for diabetic nephropathy (independent of DM and glycemic control) has not been clearly confirmed.

Smoking

Although recent studies have shown the association between smoking and progression of diabetic nephropathy, a large prospective study by Hovind et al. [70] did not confirm the association between smoking and decreased GFR rate in patients with DM with or without ACEI therapy.

Oral Contraception

Ahmed et al. [71] showed the association between the use of oral contraceptives and development of diabetic nephropathy.

Each of the above-described factors increases the risk of diabetic nephropathy, but none is predictive enough for the development of diabetic nephropathy in an individual patient.

6. Association between diabetic nephropathy and retinopathy

Patients with type 1 DM and nephropathy almost always have other complications related to the underlying disease, such as retinopathy and neuropathy [9]. Retinopathy has easily recognizable clinical manifestations and always precedes the clinically manifest signs of nephropathy in the same patient. The vice versa is not the case. A small number of patients with advanced retinopathy have glomerular histological changes and microalbuminuria, but most have no biopsy evidence of kidney disease [72]. The association between diabetic nephropathy and retinopathy is weaker in patients with type 2 DM. In a study carried out by Parving et al. [73] in 35 patients with type 2 DM and proteinuria (> 300 mg/day), 27 of these patients had biopsy evidence of nephropathy. Diabetic retinopathy was present in 15 of these 27 patients and in none of the eight patients without diabetic nephropathy. Further analysis showed that approximately one-third of patients without retinopathy had no biopsy evidence of diabetic nephropathy [74].

Thus, patients with type 2 DM and significant proteinuria and retinopathy were most likely to develop diabetic nephropathy, whereas those with proteinuria but without retinopathy had a greater likelihood of having an underlying non-diabetic kidney disease [75]. In the study by Schwartz et al, biopsy was performed in 36 patients with type 2 DM and nephropathy. In 17 of them, biopsy showed visible glomerulosclerosis with Kimmelstiel-Wilson nodules, whereas in the remaining 15 patients, biopsy showed changes characteristic of diabetic nephropathy (mesangial sclerosis), but with no classical nodules present. There was no difference in the duration of disease and glycemic regulation between patients with and those without nodules. A strong association was found between severe retinopathy and presence of Kimmelstiel-Wilson nodules. The reason is still unknown [76].

According to the K/DOQI 2007 Guidelines, etiology of kidney disease in most patients with DM should be ascribed to DM if pathologic proteinuria and retinopathy are present [77]. In case that no retinopathy is present, non-diabetic causes of kidney disease should be investigated.

7. Biomarkers of diabetic nephropaty

Albuminuria remains the only biomarker acceptable for diagnostic purposes, although some growth factors are expected to replace albuminuria in future. It is known that values of TGF beta, vascular endothelial growth factor (VEGF), and CTGF are increased in the plasma and urine of patients with diabetic nephropathy [78-80].

8. Non-diabetic kidney disease

Proteinuria is sometimes present in DM because of the primary glomerular disease rather than diabetic nephropathy. In that case, possible caused of kidney damage may include membrane nephropathy, minimal change disease, IgA nephropathy, focal glomerulosclerosis, Henoch-Schönlein purpura, proliferative glomerulonephritis, and so on. The main clinical signs of primary glomerular disease are as follows:

a. Proteinuria, which started in the first five years after the diagnosis of type 1 DM. Latent nephropathy, is present between 10 and 15 years after the onset of type 1 DM. This period is probably the same in type 2 DM, but the exact time of the onset of the disease is difficult to determine.
b. Acute onset of kidney disease. Diabetic nephropathy is a slowly developing disease.
c. The presence of erythrocytes (mostly acanthocytes) and rouleaux formations in urine sediment. Patients with microscopic hematuria may have a benign familial hematuria, which is present in approximately 9% of population with or without diabetic nephropathy [81]
d. The absence of diabetic retinopathy or neuropathy in patients with type 1 DM. As opposed to that, the absence of retinopathy in patients with type 2 DM does not exclude the presence of diabetic retinopathy.
e. Signs and/or symptoms of other systemic disease.
f. A significant decrease in GFR (>30%) within two to three months after the introduction of ACEI or angiotensin II receptor blockers (ARB) therapy.

Nephrosclerosis

Proteinuria and kidney failure in patients with DM may also be caused by other diseases apart from primary glomerular diseases. The most frequent cause is atherosclerotic vascular disease (nephrosclerosis) in older patients with type 2 DM [82]. This disease cannot be clinically discerned from diabetic nephropathy without kidney biopsy. However, kidney biopsy is not necessary in most cases, because the correct diagnosis in this patient group is not clinically important. What speaks in favor of nephrosclerosis is the significant increase in serum creatinine after the introduction of ACEI or ARB for the treatment of hypertension or slowing down the progress of chronic kidney disease. The same occurs when there is a bilateral renal artery stenosis.

9. Treatment

Strict Glycemic Control

The effect of strict glycemic control depends on the DM stage in which it was started and consequent normalization of glucose metabolism. Intensified insulin therapy has the following effects on the kidney:

a. It partly decreases glomerular hypertrophy and hyperfiltration (in fasting state and after protein-rich meal), both of which are important risk factors for permanent glomerular damage.
b. It postpones the development of albuminuria [83]. Intensified insulin therapy that keeps glucose values within normal ranges decreases the development or progress of diabetic nephropathy.

c. It stabilizes or decreases the elimination of proteins in patients with pronounced proteinuria. This effect is not apparent in patients who are not relatively normogycemic during two years. Furthermore, re-established normoglycemia after combined kidney and pancreas transplantation in patients with type 1 DM has preventive effects on recurrence of nephropathy in kidney transplant [84].
d. It slows down the progress of kidney disease in case of already developed proteinuria confirmed by semiquantitative method (test strip).
e. It reduces mesangial cell number and mesangial matrix.
f. In some patients, the thickness of glomerular and tubular basement membranes and mesangial cell number become normal and glomerular nodules disappear.
g. The progress of tubular atrophy is slowed down.

Strict Blood Pressure Control

Strict blood pressure control is important in the prevention of progress of diabetic nephropathy and other complications in patients with type 2 DM. The optimum lower range of systolic blood pressure is not clearly defined. According to the UKPDS study, a reduction in systolic blood pressure by 10 mm Hg decreases the risk of development of diabetic complications by 12%; the risk is the lowest where systolic blood pressure values are below 120 mm Hg [85]. The Irbesartan Diabetic Nephropathy Trial showed that decreasing systolic blood pressure to the lower limit value of 120 mm Hg reduces the risk of cardiovascular mortality and heart failure (but not of myocardial infarction) and the risk of double increase in serum creatinine or progress to terminal kidney failure [86].

According to the current Guidelines on Arterial Hypertension Treatment [87], the target blood pressure in patients with DM should be <130/80 mm Hg. Antihypertensive therapy may be started even when blood pressure values are in the upper normal range.

Inhibition of Renin-Angiotensin-Aldosterone System

Angiotensin II is the most effective factor of renin-angiotensin-aldosterone system (RAAS), resulting from a range of proteolytic reactions that begin with the conversion of angiotensinogen to angiotensin I through the catalytic action of renin (Figure 7).

RAAS is directly associated with blood pressure regulation, body fluid volume, and vascular response to injury and inflammation. Inappropriate activation of this system increases the blood pressure and has anti-inflammatory, prothrombotic, and proatherogenic effects, which in the long run lead to irreversible damage of target organs. Although aldosterone, renin, and end-products of angiotensin degradation are also involved in this process, majority of the RAAS effects on target organs are mediated by angiotensin II, which is present in the bloodstream and tissues. Angiotensin II, which is produced in the heart, brain, and kidneys through alternative pathways by kinase and endopeptidase activity, is more effective than angiotensin II produced in the bloodstream [88]. Angiotensin II binds to AT1 i AT2 receptors. AT1 receptor activation is responsible for vasoconstriction, release of aldosterone, vascular remodeling, oxidative stress, and has anti-inflammatory, proatherogenic, and prothrombotic effects [89]. The activation of AT2 receptors leads not

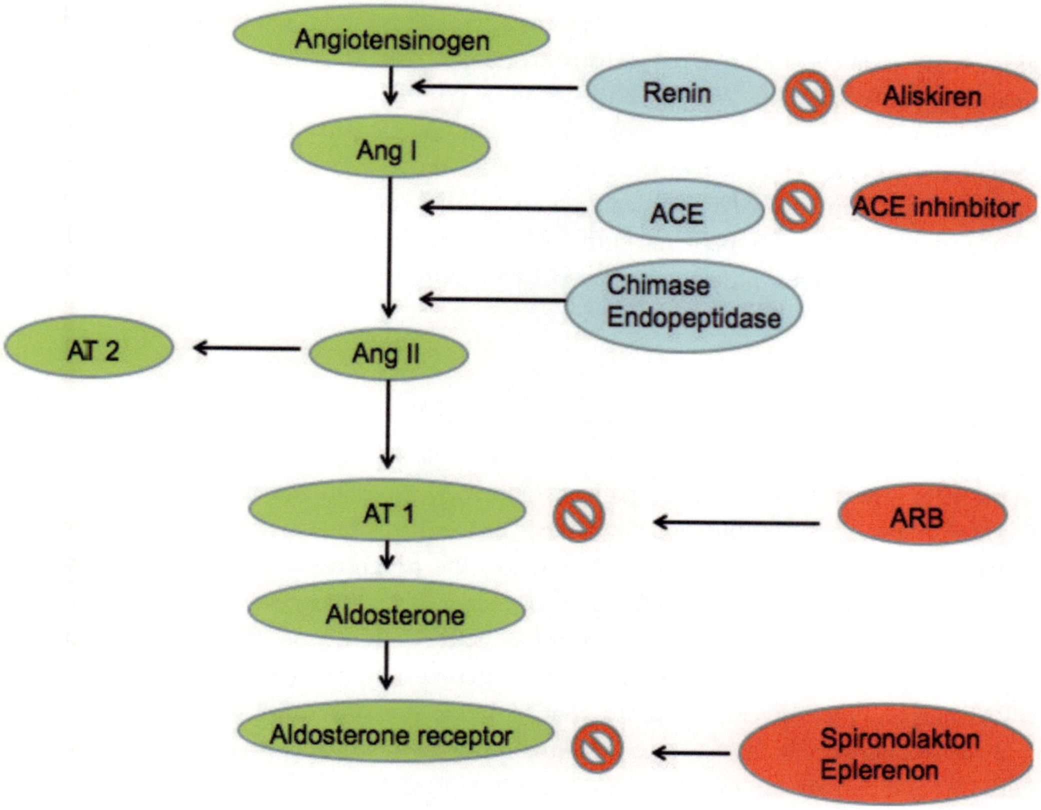

Figure 7. The RAAS and examples of RAAS inhibitors that are available for oral treatment.
ACE, angiotensin-converting enzyme; Ang I, angiotensin I; Ang II, angiotensin II; ARB, angiotensin-II-receptor blocker; AT 1, angiotensin II type 1 receptor; AT2, angiotensin II type 2 receptor; RAAS, renin-angiotensin-aldosterone system.

only to vasodilatation, growth inhibition, and antiatherogenic effects, but also to heart hypertrophy and poorer revascularization after the obstruction of coronary or peripheral artery [90]. In 1977, Ondetti et al. [91] started a new era in the research of pathophysiological role of the RAAS in kidney disease by developing the first ACEI (captopril) for the treatment of renovascular hypertension. In 1986, Zatz et al. [92] provided evidence that RAAS plays a role in the pathogenesis and progress of diabetic nephropathy by proving that enalapril decreases glomerular capillary hypertension, structural glomerular damage, and proteinuria in diabetic rats. Later studies have confirmed that angiotensin II plays the key role in the functional and structural changes linking proteinuria with the development of diabetic nephropathy. Along with pleiotropic effects, angiotensin II has effects on the structure of glomerular filtration membrane, inducing the remodeling of the podocytic cytoskeleton and causing their apoptosis, which contributes to easier ultrafiltration of plasma proteins [93]. Renoprotective effect of ACEI and ARB has been confirmed in a meta-analysis showing that ACEI and ARB decrease albuminuria in patients with DM more effectively than antihypertensive medications whose mechanism of action excludes RAAS

[94]. Early treatment with ACEI may prevent microalbuminuria, which is the early sign of glomerular damage and marker of cardiovascular risk in patients with DM. Delayed treatment with ACEI or ARB in patients with type 2 DM, diabetic nephropathy, and proteinuria is not effective enough. Increasing ACEI and ARB dosages above the recommended values for the treatment of hypertension or their combination is very effective in reducing albuminuria [95]. Aldosteron receptor antagonists and renin inhibitors also decrease albuminuria in patients with DM, but large randomized trial are needed to determine their possible advantage over ACEI and ARB either as monotherapy or combined therapy [96].

Dyslipidemia

Dyslipidemia occurs in all patients with DM, and its occurrence increases with the development of diabetic nephropathy. Aggressive plasma lipid reduction is an important therapeutic intervention, because patients with DM have an increased risk of coronary disease. In addition, dyslipidemia contributes to the development of diabetic nephropathy. Treating dyslipidemia with statins slows down the progression of diabetic nephropathy [97]. In addition to statins, fenofibrate also decreases the progression of albuminuria in patients with DM [98]. In addition to anti-inflammatory effect, it decreases the production of collagen type 1 in mesangial cells via nuclear peroxisome proliferator-activated receptors (PPAR) alpha [99]. Intensive glycemic control, blood pressure control by RAAS inhibitors, and decreasing serum lipid concentration is an optimal therapeutic approach in patients with DM and diabetic nephropathy (including the microalbuminuria stage).

The Role of Other Factors

Transforming growth factor beta (TGF-beta) has effects on cell hypertrophy and increased collagen synthesis. Inhibition of TGF-beta in experimental DM model prevented the development and progression of diabetic nephropathy [100]. Experimental studies have shown that non-dihydropyridine calcium channel blocker (diltiazem) slows down the progression of most morphological changes in diabetic nephropathy [101]. On the other hand, diltiazem monotherapy leads to the increased tubulointerstitial fibrosis and global, but not segmental, glomerulosclerosis. This negative effect of diltiazem can be corrected by ACEI therapy.

Peroxisome proliferator-activated receptors (PPAR) play a significant role in the regulation of adipogenesis, lipid metabolism, insulin sensitivity, inflammation, and blood pressure control; however, they also seem to play a significant role in the development of diabetic nephropathy in type 2 DM patients [102]. In an experimental animal model of diabetic nephropathy, PPAR gamma agonists, such as tiazolidinedones (oral hypoglicemic agents), were shown to reduce fibrosis, mesangial proliferation, and inflammation [103]. In addition, these agents reduce albuminuria in different stages of diabetic nephropathy and decrease blood pressure [104]. Their possible renoprotective effects still need to be confirmed in randomized clinical trials including a large number of patients.

New Treatment Strategies

Current treatment has not always been effective in all patients. Therefore, new treatment options are being investigated.

High doses of thiamine and its derivative benfotiamine (S-benzoylthiamine O-monophosphate) were shown to slow down the development of microalbuminuria in animal models, most likely by decreasing the activation of PKC, protein glycation, and oxidative stress [105]. In experimental animals treated with ALT-711, which metabolizes AGEs, a decrease in blood pressure and kidney damage was observed [106]. PKC-beta inhibitor (ruboxistaurin) normalizes GFR, reduces or decreases albuminuria, and improves kidney function in experimental animals [107]. Pimagedin (second generation AGE inhibitor) reduces albuminuria and GFR decrease in patients with type 1 DM and proteinuria [108].

Smaller clinical trials have produced contradictory results, while the results of large randomized clinical trials are still not available.

In an experimental model of induced glomerulosclerosis, modified heparin glycosaminoglycan prevented albuminuria, accumulation of extracellular matrix proteins, and increased expression of TGF-beta [109]. Although animal models held promise, the administration of sulodexid in a large multicentric SUN-Micro-Trial did not achieve the primary outcome, i.e., there were no significant differences in the reduction of albuminuria between the treatment and control groups [110].

10. Conclusion

In the last several years, we have witnessed an enormous progress made not only in our understanding of the risk factors and mechanism of the development of diabetic nephropathy, but also in the treatment possibilities aimed at preventing the progression of diabetic nephropathy.

Early detection of this chronic DM complication along with the treatment of main risk factors (hyperglycemia, hypertension, and dyslipidemia) and use of renoprotective drugs (ACEI and ARB) may decrease the progression of this kidney disease. The treatment of increased blood pressure is a priority. All listed measures lead to a decrease in the overall and cardiovascular mortality in patients with DM.

Author details

Božidar Vujičić and Sanjin Rački

Department of Nephrology and Dialysis, Clinical Hospital Centre Rijeka, Rijeka, Croatia

Tamara Turk and Željka Crnčević-Orlić

Department of Endocrinology, Diabetes and Metabolic Diseases, Clinical Hospital Centre Rijeka, Rijeka, Croatia

Gordana Đorđević
Department of Pathology and Pathologic Anatomy, Faculty of Medicine, University of Rijeka, Rijeka, Croatia

11. References

[1] Reutens AT, Prentice L, Atkins R (2008) The Epidemiology of Diabetic Kidney Disease, In: Ekoe J, editor. The Epidemiology of Diabetes Mellitus, 2nd Edition. Chichester: John Wiley & Sons Ltd. pp. 499-518.
[2] Adler AI, Stevens RJ, Manley SE, Bilous WR, Cull AC, Holman RR (2003) Development and progression of nephropathy in type 2 diabetes: The United Kingdom Prospective Diabetes Study (UKPDS 64). Kidney int. 225-232.
[3] Kimmelstiel P, Wilson C (1936) Benign and malignant hypertension and nephrosclerosis. A clinical and pathological study. Am. j. pathol.12:45-8.
[4] Vrhovac B, Jakšić B, Reiner Ž, Vucelić B (2008) Interna medicina. Zagreb: Naklada Ljevak. pp 1258-1259.
[5] Mogensen CE (1999) Microalbuminuria, blood presure and diabetic renal disease: origin and development of ideas. Diabetologia. 42:263-285.
[6] Buchan IE (1997) Arcus QuickStat Biomedical version. Cambridge: Addison Wesley Longman Ltd.
[7] Viberti GC, Hill RD, Jarrett RJ, Argyropoulos A, Mahmud U, Keen H (1982) Microalbuminuria as a predictor of clinical nephropathy in insulin-dependent diabetes mellitus. Lancet. 1:1430-1432.
[8] Mogensen CE (1984) Microalbuminuria predicts clinical proteinuria and early mortality in maturity-onset diabetes. New eng. j. med. 310:356-360.
[9] Orchard TJ, Dorman JS, Maser RE, Becker DJ, Drash AL, Ellis D et al. (1990) Prevalence of complications in IDDM by sex and duration. Pittsburgh Epidemiology of Diabetes Complications Study II. Diabetes. 39:1116-1124.
[10] Chaturvedi N, Bandinelli S, Mangili R, Penno G, Rottiers RE, Fuller JH (2001) Microalbuminuria in type 1 diabetes: rates, risk factors and glycemic threshold. Kidney int. 60:219-227.
[11] Hovind P, Tarnow L, Rossing P, Jensen BR, Graae M, Torp I, Binder C, Parving HH (2004) Predictors of the development of microalbuminuria and macroalbuminuria in patients with type 1 diabetes: inception cohort study. Brit. med. j. 328:1105-1108.
[12] Young BA, Maynard C, Boyko EJ (2003) Racial differences in diabetic nephropathy, cardiovascular disease, and mortality in a national population of veterans. Diabetes care. 26:2392-2399.
[13] Cowie CC, Port FK, Wolfe RA, Savage PJ, Moll PP, Hawthorne VM (1989) Disparities in incidence of diabetic end-stage renal disease according to race and type of diabetes. New engl. j. med. 321:1074-1079.
[14] Craig KJ, Donovan K, Munnery M, Owens DR, Williams JD, Phillips AO (2003) Identification and management of diabetic nephropathy in the diabetes clinic. Diabetes care. 26:1806-1811.

[15] Caramori ML, Kim Y, Huang C, Fish AJ, Rich SS, Miller ME et al. (2002) Cellular basis of diabetic nephropathy 1. Study design and renal structural-functional relationships in patients with long-standing type 1 diabetes. Diabetes. 51:506-513.

[16] Solini A, Dalla Vestra M, Saller A, Nosadini R, Crepaldi G, Fioretto P (2002) The angiotensin-converting enzyme DD genotype is associated with glomerulopathy lesions in type 2 diabetes. Diabetes. 51:251-255.

[17] Rudberg S, Rasmussen LM, Bangstad HJ, Osterby R (2000) Influence of insertion/deletion polymorphism in the ACE-I gene on the progression of diabetic glomerulopathy in type 1 diabetic patients with microalbuminuria. Diabetes care. 23:544-8.

[18] Harris RD, Steffes MW, Bilous RW, Sutherland DER, Mauer SM (1991) Global glomerular sclerosis and glomerular arteriolar hyalinosis in insulin dependent diabetes. Kidney int. 40:107-114.

[19] Olson JL, de Urdaneta AG, Heptinstall RH (1985) Glomerular hyalinosis and its relation to hyperfiltration. Lab. invest.52:387-398.

[20] Ruggenenti P, Gambara V, Perna A, Bertani T, Remuzzi G (1998) The nephropathy of non-insulin-dependent diabetes: Predictors of outcome relative to diverse patterns of renal injury. J. am. soc. nephrol. 9:2336-2343.

[21] Reddy GR, Kotlyarevska K, Ransom RF, Menon RK (2008) The podocyte and diabets mellitus: is the podocyte the key to the origins of diabetic nephropathy? Curr. opin. nephrol. hypertens.17:32-36.

[22] Tervaert TWC, Mooyaart AL, Amann K, Cohen AH, Cook HT, Drachenberg CB et al. on behalf of the Renal pathology Society (2010) Pathologic Classification of Diabetic Nephropathy. J. am. soc. nephrol. 21:556-563.

[23] Nasr SH, D'Agati VD (2007) Nodular glomerulosclerosis in the nondiabetic smoker. J. am. soc. nephrol. 18:2032-2036.

[24] Olsen S, Mogensen CE (1996) How often is NIDDM complicated with non-diabetic renal disease? An analysis of renal biopsies and the literature. Diabetologia. 39:1638-1645.

[25] Galesic K, Sabljar-Matovinovic M, Prkacin I, Kovacević-Vojtusek I (2009) Dijabeticka nefropatija i primarne bolesti glomerula. Lijec. vjesn. 131:141-145.

[26] Stadler G, Schmidt R (1959) Severe funcional disorders of glomerular capillaries and renal hemodynamics in treated diabetes mellitus during childhood. Ann. pediatr. 193:129-138.

[27] Mogensen CE (1971) Kidney function and glomerular permeability to macromolecules in early juvenile diabetes. Scand. j. clin. lab. invest. 28:79-90.

[28] Serri O, Beauregard H, Brazeau P, Aribat T, Lambert J, Harris A et al. (1991) Somatostatin analogue, octreotide, reduces increased glomerular filtration rate and kidney size in insulin-dependent diabetics. JAMA. 265:888-892.

[29] Hirschberg R, Brunori G, Kopple JD, Guler, HP (1993) Effects of insulin-like growth factor I on renal function in normal men. Kidney int. 43:387-397.

[30] Hirschberg R, Kopple JD (1992) The growth hormone-insulin-like growth factor I axis and renal glomerular filtration. J. am. soc. nephrol. 2:1417-1422.

[31] Cherney DZ, Sochett EB, Miller JA (2005) Gender differences in renal responses to hyperglycemia and angiotensin-converting enzyme inhibition in diabetes. Kidney int. 68:1722-1728.
[32] Passariello N, Sepe J, Marrazzo G, De Cicco A, Peluso A, Pisano MC et al. (1993) Effect of aldose reductase inhibitor (tolrestat) on urinary albumin excretion rate and glomerular filtration rate in IDDM subjects with nephropathy. Diabetes care. 16:789-795.
[33] Vallon V, Blantz RC, Thomson S (2003) Glomerular hyperfiltration and the salt paradox in rarely type 1 diabetes mellitus: a tubulo-centric view. J. am. soc. nephrol. 14:530-537.
[34] Vallon V, Richter K, Blantz RC, Thomson S, Osswald H (1999) Glomerular hyperfiltration in experimental diabetes mellitus: Potential role of tubular reabsorption. J. am. soc. nephrol. 10:2569-2576.
[35] Vlassara H. Protein glycation in the kidney: Role in diabetes and aging (1996) Kidney int. 49:1795-1804.
[36] Zhou G, Li C, Cai L (2004) Advanced glycation end-products induce connective tissue growth factor –mediated renal fibrosis predominately through transforming growth factor beta-independent pathway. Am. j. pathol. 165:2033-2043.
[37] Sabbatini M, Sansone G, Uccello F, Giliberti A, Conte G, Andreucci VE (1992) Early glycosilation products induce glomerular hyperfiltration in normal rats. Kidney int. 42:875-881.
[38] Heilig CW, Concepcion LA, Riser BL, Freytag SO, Zhu M, Cortes P (1995) Overexpression of glucose transporters in mesangial cells cultured in a normal glucos milieu mimics the diabetic phenotype. J. clin. invest. 96:1802-1814.
[39] Lin CL, Wang JY, Huang YT, Kuo YH, Surendran K, wang FS (2006) Wnt/beta-catenin signaling modulates survival of high glucose-stressed mesangial cells. J. am. soc. nephrol. 17:2812-2820.
[40] Cooper ME (1998) Pathogenesis, prevention, and treatment of diabetic nephropathy. Lancet. 352:213-219.
[41] van den Hoven MJ, Rops AL, Bakker MA, Aten J, Rutjes N, Roestenberg P et.al. (2006) Increased expression of heparanase in overt diabetic nephropathy. Kidney int. 70:2100-2108.
[42] Dronavalli S, Duka I, Bakris GL (2008) The pathogenesis of diabetic nephropathy. Nat. clin. pract. endocrinol. metab. 4:444-4452.
[43] Daneman D, Crompton CH, Balfe JW, Sochett EB, Chatzilias A, Cotter BR et.al. (1994) Plasma prorenin as an early marker of nephropathy in diabetic (IDDM) adolescents. Kidney int. 46:1154-1159.
[44] Nguyen G (2006) Renin/prorenin receptors. Kidney int. 69:1503-1506.
[45] Ichihara A, Suzuki F, Nakagawa T, Kaneshiro Y, Takemitsu T, Sakoda M et.al. (2006) Prorenin receptor blockade inhibits development of glomerulosclerosis in diabetic angiotensin II type 1a receptor-deficient mice. J. am. soc. nephrol. 17:1950-1961.
[46] Hohenstein B, Hausknecht B, Boehmer K, Riess R, Brekken RA, Hugo CPM (2006) Local VEGF activity but not VEGF expression is tightly regulated during diabetic nephropathy in man. Kidney int. 69:1654-1661.
[47] Navarro-Gonzalez JF, Mora-Fernandez C (2008) The role of inflammatory cytokines in diabetic nephropathy. J. am. soc. nephrol. 19:433-442.

[48] Langham RG, Kelly DJ, Maguire J, Dowling JP, Gilbert RE, Thomson NM (2003) Over-expression of platelet-derived growth factor in human diabetic nephropathy. Nephrol. dial. transplant. 18:1392-1396.

[49] Wolf G, Ziyadeh FN. Molecular mechanisms of diabetic renal hypertrophy (1999) Kidney int. 56:393-405.

[50] Wang S, de Caestecker M, Kopp J, Mitu G, LaPage J, Hirschberg R (2006) Renal bone morphogenetic protein-7 protects against diabetic nephropathy. J. am. soc. nephrol. 17:2504-2512.

[51] Turk T, Leeuwis JW, Gray J, Torti SV, Lyons KM, Nguyen TQ et al. (2009) BMP signaling and podocyte markers are decreased in human diabetic nephropathy in association with CTGF overexpression. J. histochem. cytochem. 57:623-631.

[52] Langham RG, Kelly DJ, Cox AJ, Thomson NM, Holthöfer H, Zaoui P et al. (2002) Proteinuria and the expression of the podocyte slit diaphragm protein, nephrin, in diabetic nephropathy: effects of angiotensin converting enzyme inhibition. Diabetologia. 45:1572-1576.

[53] Tap RJ, Shaw JE, Zimmet PZ, Balkau B, Chadban SJ, Tonkin AM et al. (2004) Albuminuria is evident in the early stages of diabetes onset: results from the Australian Diabetes, Obesity, and Lifestyle Study (AusDiab). Am. j. kidney dis. 44:792-798.

[54] Satko SG, Langefeld CD, Daeihagh P, Bowden DB, Rich SS, Freedman BI (2002) Nephropathy in siblings of African Americans with overt type 2 diabetic nephropathy. Am. j. kidney dis. 40:489-494.

[55] Brancati FL, Whittle JC, Whelton PK, Seidler AJ, Klag MJ (1992) The excess incidence of diabetic end-stage renal disease among blacks. A population-based study of potential explanatory factors. JAMA. 268:3079-3084.

[56] Svensson M, Nystrom L, Schon S, Dahlquist G (2006) Age at onset of childhood-onset type 1 diabetes and the development of end-stage renal disease: a nationwide population-based study. Diabetes care. 29:538-542.

[57] Patel A: ADVANCE Collaborative Group (2007) Effects of a fixed combination of perindopril and indapamide on macrovascular and microvascular outcomes in patients with type 2 diabetes mellitus (the ADVANCE trial): a randomised controlled trial. Lancet. 370:829-840.

[58] Randeree HA, Omar MA, Motala AA, Seedat MA (1992) Effect of insulin therapy on blood pressure in NIDDM patients with secondary failure. Diabetes care. 15:1258-1263.

[59] Nosadini R, Sambataro M, Thomaseth K, Pacini G, Cipollina MR, Brocco E et al. (1993) Role of hyperglycemia and insulin resistance in determining sodium retention in non-insulin-dependent diabetes. Kidney int. 44:139-146.

[60] Cruickshank K, Riste L, Anderson SG, Wright JS, Dunn G, Gosling RG (2002) Aortic pulse-wave velocity and its relationship to mortality in diabetes and glucose intolerance: an integrated index of vascular function? Circulation. 106:2085-2090.

[61] Pavkov Me, Bennett PH, Knowler WC, Krakoff J, Sievers ML, Nelson RG (2006) Effect of youth-onset type 2 diabetes mellitus on incidence of end-stage renal disease and mortality in young and middle-aged Pima Indians. JAMA. 296:421-426.

[62] Tuttle KR, Bruton JL, Perusek MC, Lancaster JL, Kopp DT, DeFronzo RA (1991) Effect of strict glycemic control on renal hemodynamic response to amino acids and renal enlargement in insulin-dependent diabetes mellitus. N. engl. j. med. 324:1626-1632.

[63] Vora JP, Dolben J, Dean JD, Thomas D, Williams JD, Owens DR et al. (1992) Renal hemodynamics in newly presenting non-insulin dependent diabetes mellitus. Kidney int. 41:829-835.

[64] Gambara V, Mecca G, Remuzzi G, Bertani T (1993) Heterogeneous nature of renal lesions in type II diabetes. J. am. soc. nephrol. 3:1458-1466.

[65] Earle K, Viberti GC (1994) Familial, hemodynamic and metabolic factors in the predisposition to diabetic kidney disease. Kidney int. 45:434-437.

[66] Hayashi K, Epstein M, Loutzenheiser R, Forster H (1992) Impaired myogenic responsiveness of afferent arteriole in streptozotocin-induced diabetic rats: Role of eicosanoid derangements. J. am. soc. nephrol. 2:1578-1586.

[67] Bash LD, Selvin E, Steffes M, Coresh J, Astor BC (2008) Poor glycemic control in diabetes and the risk of incident chronic kidney disease even in the absence of albuminuria and retinopathy: Atherosclerosis Risk in Communities (ARIC) Study. Arch. intern. med. 168:2440-2447.

[68] Krolewski M, Eggers PW, Warram JH (1996) Magnitude of end stage renal disease in IDDM: A 35 year follow-up study. Kidney int. 50:2041-2046.

[69] Saiki A, Nagayama D, Ohhira M, Endoh K, Ohtsuka M, Koide N et al. (2005) Effect of weight loss using formula diet on renal function in obese patients with diabetic nephropathy. Int. j. obes. 29:1115-1120.

[70] Hovind P, Rossing P, Tarnow L, Parving HH (2003) Smoking and progression of diabetic nephropathy in type 1 diabetes. Diabetes care. 26:911-916.

[71] Ahmed SB, Hovind P, Parving HH, Rossing P, Price DA, Laffel LM et al. (2005) Oral contraceptives, angiotensin-dependent renal vasoconstriction, and risk of diabetic nephropathy. Diabetes care. 28:1988-1994.

[72] Chavers BM, Mauer SM, Ramsay RC, Steffes MW (1994) Relationship between retinal and glomerular lesions in IDDM patients. Diabetes. 43:441-446.

[73] Parving HH, Gall MA, Skott P, Jorgensen HE, Lokkegaard H, Jorgensen F et al. (1992) Prevalence and causes of albuminuria in non-insulin-dependent diabetic patients. Kidney int. 41:758-762.

[74] Christensen PK, Larsen S, Horn T, Olsen S, Parving HH (2000) Causes of albuminuria in patients with type 2 diabetes without diabetic retinopathy. Kidney int. 58:1719-1731.

[75] Huang F, Yang Q, Chen L, Tang S, Liu W, Yu X (2007) Renal pathological change in patients with type 2 diabetes is not always diabetic nephropathy: a report of 52 cases. Clin. nephrol. 67:293-297.

[76] Schwartz MM, Lewis EJ, Leonard-Martin T, Lewis JB, Batlle D (1998) Renal pathology patterns in type II diabetes mellitus: Relationship with retinopathy. Nephrol. dial. transplant. 13:2547-2552.

[77] K/DOQI clinical practice guidelines and clinical practice recommendations for diabetes and chronic kidney disease (2007) Am. j. kidney dis. 49:S12.

[78] Nguyen TQ, Tarnow L, Jorsal A, Oliver N, Roestenberg P, Ito Y et al. (2008) Plasma connective tissue growth factor is an independent predictor of end-stage renal disease and mortalityin type 1 diabetic nephropathy. Diabetes care. 31:1177-1182.

[79] Nguyen TQ, Tarnow L, Andersen S, Hovind P, Parvinh HH, Goldschmeding R et al. (2006) Urinary connective tissue growth factor excretion correlates with clinical markers

of renal disease in a large population of type 1 diabetic patients with diabetic nephropathy. Diabetes care. 29:83-88.

[80] Pfeiffer A, Middelberg-Bisping K, Drewes C, Shatz H (1996) Elevated plasma levels of transforming growth factor-beta 1 in NIDDM. Diabetes care. 19:1113-1117.

[81] Heine GH, Sester U, Girndt M, Kohler H (2004) Acanthocytes in the urine: useful tool to differentiate diabetic nephropathy from glomerulonephritis?. Diabetes care. 27:190-194.

[82] Myers DI, Poole LJ, Imam K, Scheel PJ, Eustace JA (2003) Renal artery stenosis by three-dimensional magnetic resonance angiography in type 2 diabetics with uncontrolled hypertension and chronic renal insufficiency: Prevalence and effect on renal function. Am. j. kidney dis. 41:351-359.

[83] Writing Team for the Diabetes Control and Complications Trial/Epidemiology of Diabetes Interventions and Complications Research Group. Sustained effect of intensive treatment of type 1 diabetes mellitus on development and progression of diabetic nephropathy: the Epidemiology of Diabetes Interventions and Complications (EDIC) study (2003) JAMA. 290:2159-2167.

[84] Fioretto P, Sutherland DE, Najafian B, Mauer M (2006) Remodeling of renal interstitial and tubular lesions in pancreas transplant recipients. Kidney int. 69:907-912.

[85] Ferrario CM (2006) Role of angiotensin II in cardiovascular disease therapeutic of more than a century of research. J. renin angiotensin aldosterone syst. 7:3-14.

[86] Berl T, Hunsicker LG, Lewis JB, Pffefer MA, Porush JG, Rouleau JL et al. (2005) Impact of achieved blood pressure on cardiovascular outcomes in the irbesartan diabetic nephropathy trial. J. am. soc. nephrol. 16:2170-2179.

[87] European Society of Hypertension (2007) Guidelines for the Management of Arterial Hypertension. J. of hyperten. 25:1105-1187.

[88] Cooper ME (2004) The role of the renin-angiotenzin-aldosterone system in diabetes and its vascular complications. Am. j. hypertens. 17:16-20.

[89] Hilgers KF, Mann JF (2002) ACE inhibitors versus AT(1) receptor antagonists in patients with chronic renal disease. J. am. soc. nephrol. 13:1100-1108.

[90] Reudelhuber TL (2005) The continuing saga of the AT2 receptor: a case of the good, the bad, and the innocuous. Hypertension. 46:1261-1262.

[91] Ondetti MA, Rubin B, Cushman DW (1977) Design of specific inhibitors of angiotensin-converting enzyme: new class of orally active antihypertensive agents. Science. 196:441-444.

[92] Zatz R, Dunn BR, Meyer TW, Anderson S, Rennke HG, Brenner BM (1986) Prevention of diabetic glomerulopathy by pharmacological amelioration of glomerular capillary hypertension. J. clin. invest. 77:1925-1930.

[93] Perico N, Benigni A, Remuzzi G (2008) Present and future drug treatments for chronic kidney disease: evolving targets in renoprotection. Nat. rev. drug. discov. 7:936-953.

[94] Casas J, Chua W, Loukogeorgakis S, Vallance P, Smeeth L, Hingorani A et al. (2005) Effect of inhibitors of the renin-angiotensin system and other antihypertensive drugs on renal outcomes: systematic review and meta-analysis. Lancet. 366:2026-2033.

[95] Jacobsen P, Andersen S, Rossing K, Jensen BR, Parving HH (2003) Dual blockade of the renin-angiotensin system versus maximal recommended dose of ACE inhibition in diabetic nephropathy. Kidney int. 63:1874-1880.

[96] Estacio RO (2009) Renin-angiotensin-aldosterone system blockade in diabetes: role of direct renin inhibitors. Postgrad. med. 121:33-44.
[97] Tonolo G, Velussi M, Brocco E, Abaterusso C, Carro A, Morgia G et al. (2006) Simvastatin maintains steady patterns of GFR and improves AER and expression of slit diaphragm proteins in type II diabetes. Kidney int. 70:177-186.
[98] Ansquer JC, Foucher C, Rattier S, Taskinen MR, Steiner G (2005) Fenofibrate reduces progression to microalbuminuria over 3 years in a placebo-controlled study in type 2 diabetes: results from the Diabetes Atherosclerosis Intervention Study (DAIS). Am. j. kidney dis. 45:485-493.
[99] Park CW, Zhang Y, Zhang X, Wu J, Chen L, Cha DR et al. (2006) PPARalpha agonist fenofibrate improves diabetic nephropathy in db/db mice. Kidney int. 69:1511-1517.
[100] Benigni A, Zoja C, Corna D, Zatelli C, Conti S, Campana M (2003) Add On Anti-TGF-β Antobody to ACE Inhibitor Arrests Progressive Diabetic Nephropathy in the Rat. J. am. soc. nephrol. 14:1816-1824.
[101] Gaber L, Walton C, Brown S, Bakris G (1994) Effects of different antihypertensive treatments on morphologic progression of diabetic nephropathy in uninephrectomized dogs. Kidney int. 46:161-169.
[102] Guan Y (2004) Peroxisome proliferator-activated receptor family and its relationship to renal complications of the metabolic syndrome. J. am. soc. nephrol. 15:2801-2815.
[103] Weissgarten J, Berman S, Efrati S, Rapaport M, Averbukh Z, Feldman L (2006) Apoptosis and proliferation of cultured mesangial cells isolated from kidneys of rosiglitazone-treated pregnant diabetic rats. Nephrol. dial. transplant. 21:1198-1204.
[104] Bakris GL, Ruilope LM, McMorn SO, Weston WM, Heise MA, Freed MI et al. (2006) Rosiglitazone reduces microalbuminuria and blood pressure independently of glycemia in type 2 diabetes patients with microalbuminuria. J. hypertens. 24:2047-2055.
[105] Babaei-Jadidi R, Karachalias N, Ahmed N, Battah S, Thornalley PJ (2003) Prevention of incipient diabetic nephropathy by high-dose thiamine and benfotiamine. Diabetes. 52:2110–2120.
[106] Forbes JM, Thallas V, Thomas MC, Founds HW, Burns WC, Jerums G et al. (2003) The breakdown of preexisting advanced glycation end products is associated with reduced renal fibrosis in experimental diabetes. FASEB j. 17:1762–1764.
[107] Kelly DJ, Zhang Y, Hepper C, Gow RM, Jaworski K, Kemp BE et al. (2003) Protein kinase C β inhibition attenuates the progression of experimental diabetic nephropathy in the presence of continued hypertension. Diabetes. 52:512–518.
[108] Bolton WK, Cattran DC, Williams ME, Adler SG, Appel GB, Cartwright K et al. (2004) Randomized trial of an inhibitor of formation of advanced glycation end products in diabetic nephropathy. Am. j. nephrol. 24:32–40.
[109] Ceol M, Gambaro G, Sauer U, Baggio B, Anglani F, Forino M et al. (2000) Glycosaminoglycan therapy prevents TGF-beta1 overexpression and pathologic changes in renal tissue of long-term diabetic rats. J. am. soc. nephrol. 11:2324-2336.
[110] Burney BO, Kalaitzidis RG, Bakris GL (2009) Novel therapies of diabetic nephropathy. Curr. opin. nephrol. hypertens. 18:107-111.

Chapter 5

Wavelet Image Fusion Approach for Classification of Ultrasound Placenta Complicated by Gestational Diabetes Mellitus

G. Malathi and V. Shanthi

Additional information is available at the end of the chapter

http://dx.doi.org/10.5772/53530

1. Introduction

The steady increase in population correspondingly increases the number of diseases people are prone to. The early diagnosis of a disease is of paramount importance, which is a major challenge faced by the medical experts. Health information, especially, clinical information increases on a daily basis and is extremely variable and is also complicate to assess. As a result, there is a demand for finding the criteria that can be used to evaluate the quality of hidden information. One of the most important problems of medical diagnosis, in general, is the subjectivity of the specialist. All these factors have resulted in the use of computers to assist the experts in their diagnosis.

Computer assisted information retrieval may assist to support quality decision making and avoid human error. Although human decision-making is often optimal, it is poor when huge amounts of data are involved for classification. Computer Aided Diagnosis (CAD) is a fast growing research field that has set a new horizon in the medical domain. It has increased the quality of current medical imaging technologies by bringing in new developments in medical imaging technology. CAD has already been successfully implemented for a number of medical problems which includes cancer, fractures etc. Even though CAD software's were developed for uncovering many diseases like microcalcification in mammograms, chest, colon, brain, liver, skeletal and vascular systems, is lacking application to ultrasound obstetrics and gynecology domain.

The human placenta is a fetus's lifeline during gestation, providing nutrients and antibodies, while eliminating waste products via the mother's blood supply. The placenta is an integral part of the child's development, but is generally disposed of, after delivery. The relatively new field of placenta analysis within the field of prenatal pathology investigates the possibility of learning important health information about the fetus from the placenta. The general opinion on the placenta is its use in the exaction of stem cells. Beyond that the placenta holds vital information that can contribute to clinical practice and the growth of the fetus in the womb. The placenta is connected to the uterine wall and exchanges nutrients and waste through the placental blood barrier. The Figure 1 represents the human placenta [1] during the pregnancy.

Gestational Diabetes or Gestational Diabetes Mellitus (GDM) is a condition in which women without previously diagnosed diabetes exhibit high blood glucose levels during pregnancy.

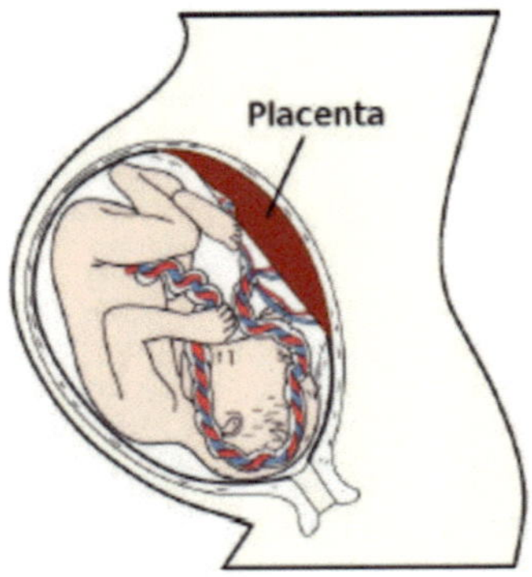

Figure 1. Placenta and fetus during pregnancy

About 80% of the diabetes [2-3] in the world will be present in developing countries like India. India accounts for the largest number of people, about 50.8 million [4] suffering from diabetes in the world, followed by China with about 43.2 million and the United States with 26.8 million, as per the new figures released by the International Diabetes Federation in the year 2009. As per the reports of World Health Organization [5], the number of diabetics throughout the world was 171 million in the year 2000 and expected to reach 350 million by 2030. The diagnosis of GDM is an important public health issue. Gestational diabetes is much more common than pre-existing [6] diabetes as it complicates about 2-5% of pregnancies.

Gestational diabetes is formally defined as "any degree of glucose intolerance with onset or first recognition during pregnancy". Gestational diabetes is caused when the body of a pregnant women does not secrete excess insulin [7] required during pregnancy leading to increased sugar levels. This definition acknowledges the possibility that patients may have previously undiagnosed diabetes mellitus or may have developed diabetes [8] coincidentally with pregnancy. Babies born to mothers with gestational diabetes are typically at increased risk of problems such as being large for gestational age.

A random survey by a team of doctors under Dr.V.Seshiah (Diabetes Care and Research Institute) showed [9] a statistics (2002) that about 16.2% of pregnant women in Chennai were found to have GDM.

Screening examinations during pregnancy are an essential part of prenatal care. Among the various screening tests that are now offered to pregnant women, ultrasound has the broadest diagnostic spectrum. There is no modality that can detect as many abnormalities [10] throughout pregnancy as ultrasound. Another important advantage of ultrasound is its low cost. Besides the early detection of a nonviable pregnancy ultrasound at the end of the first trimester can detect gross fetal anomalies or at least show initial signs that are suggestive of complications. The examination of the placenta appears to be treated with less attention than the fetus or the pregnant uterus. A methodical sonographic evaluation of the placenta plays a foremost role in the assessment of normal and abnormal pregnancies.

There are different ways in which the ultrasound [11] technology can be used in pregnancy related diagnosis.

- Abdominal ultrasound: Abdominal Ultrasound is the most common used in pregnancy related diagnosis. In this ultrasound the sonologists moves the transducer over the abdomen to scan the uterus and examine the development of the baby and several other conditions of the uterus. This research uses ultrasound images of placenta obtained by abdominal scan.
- Vaginal Ultrasound: In vaginal ultrasound, a sterilized probe is gently placed in the vagina but outside the cervix. The probe is covered with a thin plastic sheath. This technique helps sonologists to minutely observe the women's uterus.
- Doppler Ultrasound: Doppler ultrasound is used to examine the blood flow in the vessels. This technique is performed in the same way as abdominal ultrasound.

Placental development is a complex process of various coordinated differentiation steps that are mostly completed at the end of the second trimester. Thereafter, placental growth is predominantly characterized by mass expansion. Thus, development of placenta precedes fetal development and growth, the latter being pronounced in the third trimester. Any increase of the diabetes in maternal environment during the critical period of placental differentiation during the first and second trimester, introduces changes in the placenta morphology which has a profound effect on subsequent fetal growth and this is the focus point of this research. The human placenta undergoes a number of structural [12] changes which ultimately will facilitate the development of the fetus. A novel study [13] conducted in Tamil Nadu by a team of doctors in the year 2012 suggested the screening of pregnant women for gestational diabetes as early as at 16 weeks of gestation.

The number of women affected [14-15] by GDM is 3 to 10% of pregnancies. Certain factors that contribute to placental abruption [16] are women having gestational diabetes and preeclampsia. The miscarriages of 44% and neural tube defects occur thirteen to twenty times more frequently in diabetic [15] pregnancy.

Placental volumes vary in dimensions depending on the ethnic backgrounds of women universally. Taking into consideration of this vital factor, the present study focuses on the Dravidian race, a sub-division of the great Negroid race. The Caucasian, Mongoloid and Australoid races exhibit different qualities of placental characteristics and are beyond the scope of the present research.

The need of this study is to evaluate the effect of GDM on the development of placental growth. Diabetic pregnancy shows increase in the size of the placenta. This affects the growth of the fetus, which may even lead to death if untreated. The evaluation of the volume of placenta at fifteen to twenty weeks of gestation can identify placenta complicated by diabetes mellitus. This would help to diagnose complications at the earliest, which would minimize the loss, birth defects and placenta abruption. Considering the placenta, size alone may be sufficient to identify a subset of women at a higher risk in the initial ultrasound examination. An increase or decrease in the size of the placenta is a strong indication to an approaching complication in the placenta. The gestational age can be prolonged only if the problem in the placenta is identified in the initial phases of pregnancy.

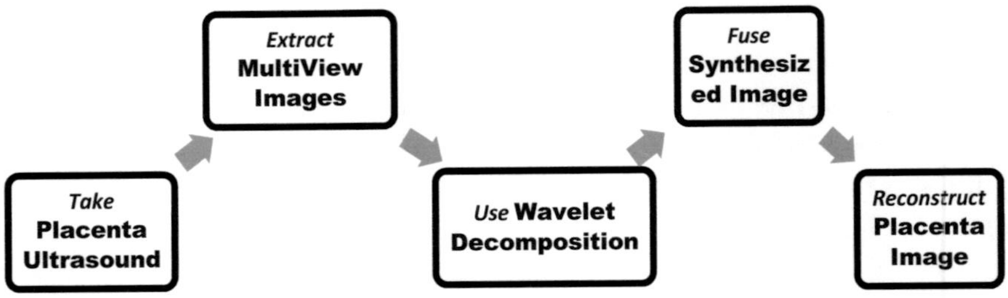

Figure 2. Approach to Decompose and Reconstruct the Fused Ultrasound Placenta from Multi-View Image Fusion

The ultrasound images of placenta obtained from the B-mode ultrasound scanner is usually low in resolution. The characteristic feature of the placenta, which plays an important role in classification, is lost because of poor resolution. There is a need for a technique to retain the finer details of the placenta in the ultrasound. In this research, the multi-view placenta images (transverse scans of placenta ultrasound images captured at the right and left of the monitor) are subjected to wavelet decomposition. The essential attribute of the ultrasound placenta is retained, when wavelet- decomposition is employed, since it is an efficient tool to extract the features of an image. When an ultrasound placenta is subjected to wavelet decomposition, the image is decomposed into different frequencies. The prominent features in these frequencies are fused into a synthesized image.

2. Why prefer wavelet?

Any decomposition of an image into wavelets involves a pair of waveforms. These represent the high frequencies corresponding to the detailed parts of an image called as wavelet function. The other represent low frequencies or smooth parts of an image called scaling function. The principle of the wavelet decomposition is to transform the original raw image into several components with single low-resolution component called "approximation" and the other components called "details" as shown in Figure 3. The approximation component is obtained after applying bi-orthogonal low-pass wavelet in each direction i.e. horizontal and vertical followed by a sub-sampling of each image by a factor of two for each dimension

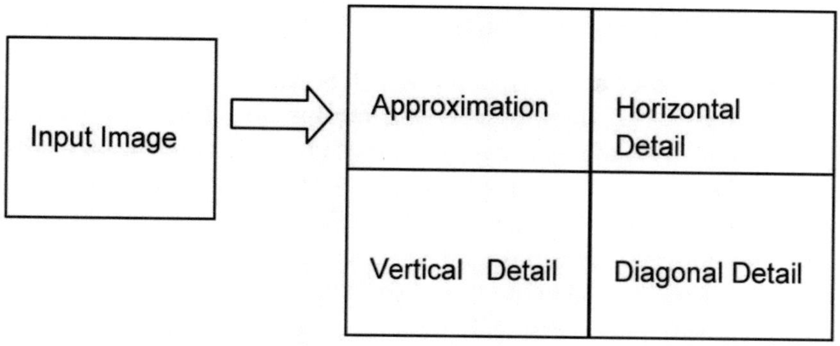

Figure 3. Wavelet Decomposition of a 2D Image

The details are obtained with the application of low-pass filter in one direction and a high-pass in the other or a high-pass in both the directions. The noise is mainly present in the details components. A higher level of decomposition is obtained by repeating the same operations on the approximation. For small details it is not obvious to a non-expert in the diagnosis of ultrasound images to know what is needed to eliminate or to preserve and enhance.

The horizontal edges of the original image are present in the horizontal detail coefficients of the upper-right quadrant. The vertical edges of the image can be similarly identified in the vertical detail coefficients of the lower-left quadrant. To combine this information into a single edge image, we simply zero the approximation coefficients of the generated transform. Compute the inverse of it and obtain the absolute value.

The images are considered to be matrices with N rows and M columns. At every level of decomposition the horizontal data is filtered, and then the approximation and details produced from this are filtered on columns. At every level, four sub images are obtained, the approximation, the vertical detail, the horizontal detail and the diagonal detail. The next level of decomposition can be obtained by the decomposition of approximation sub-image. The multilevel decomposition of an image is given in Figure 4.

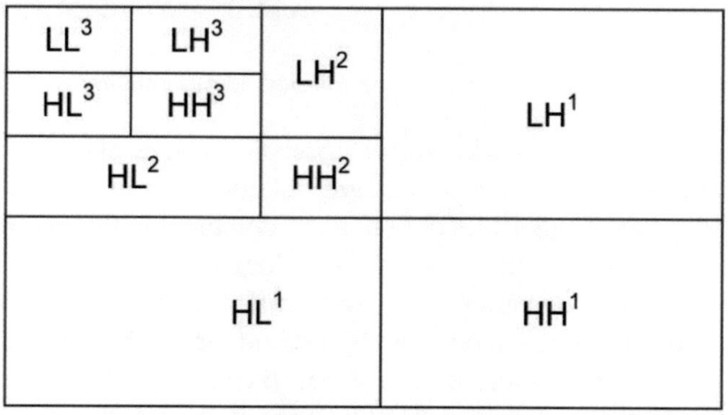

Figure 4. Multilevel Wavelet Decomposition of an Image

2.1. Choice of mother wavelet

The choice of wavelet bases depends on the signal. Signals coming from different sources have different characteristics. The wavelet basis functions are obtained from a single mother wavelet by translation and scaling. However, there is no single or universal mother wavelet function. The mother wavelet must simply satisfy a small set of conditions and is typically selected based on the domain of the signal or image processing problem. The best choices of wavelet bases are not clear for ultrasound placenta images. The problem is to represent typical signals with a small number of convenient computable functions. An investigation to choose the best wavelet for ultrasound images was performed on ultrasound placenta image. The majority of the wavelet bases which exist in the Matlab 7 version software were tested. The Haar wavelet is chosen for the decomposition of ultrasound placenta images. Higher levels of decomposition showed promising diagnostic features of the ultrasound placenta image.

2.2. Haar wavelet decomposition of ultrasound placenta

Haar wavelet basis can be used to represent an image by computing a wavelet transform. The pixel is averaged together pair-wise and is calculated to obtain the new resolution image with pixel values. Some information may be lost in the averaging process. The Haar wavelet transform is used to analyze images effectively and efficiently at various resolutions. It is used to get the approximation coefficients and detail coefficients at various levels.

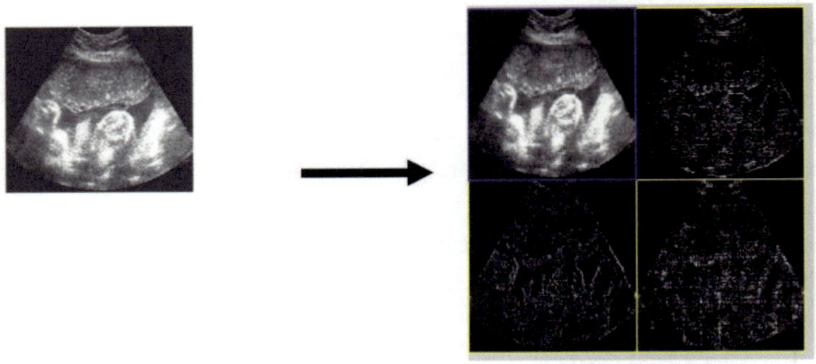

Figure 5. Level-1 Haar Wavelet Decomposition of an ultrasound placenta image

The ultrasound images of placenta with various gestational ages like 10 weeks, 12 weeks, 15 weeks, 17 weeks, and greater than 20 weeks are obtained from Chennai based Diagnostic Scan Centers. The placenta images thus obtained are demarcated into a normal placenta and GDM complicated placenta with the help of the sonologists. These images are then subjected to different levels of wavelet decomposition using different wavelets. The transverse scans of placenta are captured with differences of few seconds from the same mother. The multi-view ultrasound placenta is subjected to various levels (1, 2, 3 and 4) of wavelet decomposition. The synthesized image of the input image is obtained as a result. This synthesized image only forms the basis to image fusion in the sections that follows. The decomposition is done to extract the useful features from the multiview placenta. Still, these images cannot be used unless a quality assessment is done. To ensure the diagnostic accuracy of the images, quality evaluation metrics are used to evaluate the performance of the wavelets. The following Figure 5 is the representation of level-1 decomposition of ultrasound placenta using Haar.

Each of the transverse and longitudinal scans of the ultrasound placenta image is decomposed into approximate, horizontal, vertical and diagonal details. N levels of decomposition can be done. Here, 4-levels of decomposition are used. The multilevel decomposition of ultrasound placenta using Haar Wavelet is represented in the Figure 6. After that, quantization is done on the decomposed image where different quantization may be done on different components thus maximizing the amount of required details and ignoring the redundant details. In order to decide the most appropriate wavelet function for the ultrasound placenta, the image is decomposed using various wavelet functions. The wavelet function is chosen based on the results of image fusion quality measures.

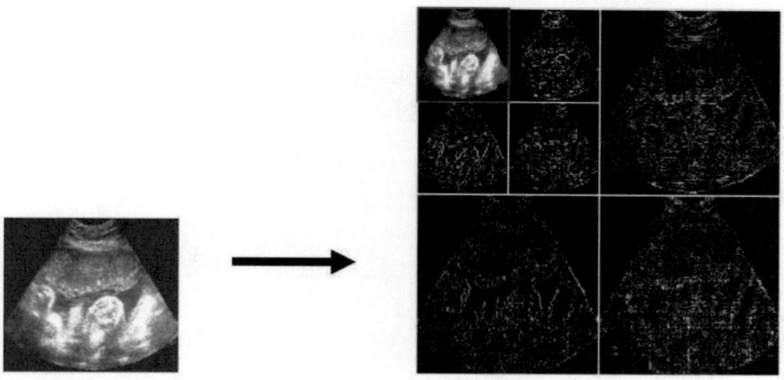

Figure 6. Multilevel Decomposition of Ultrasound Placenta using Haar Wavelet

The Figure 7 gives the synthesized ultrasound images of placenta obtained from Haar, Daubechies and Symlet wavelet decomposition. The Haar wavelet is chosen in this research because of its good entropy and mutual information. However, the fact that they have dump discontinuities in particular in the poorly decaying Haar coefficients of smooth functions and the images reconstructed from subsets of the Haar coefficients.

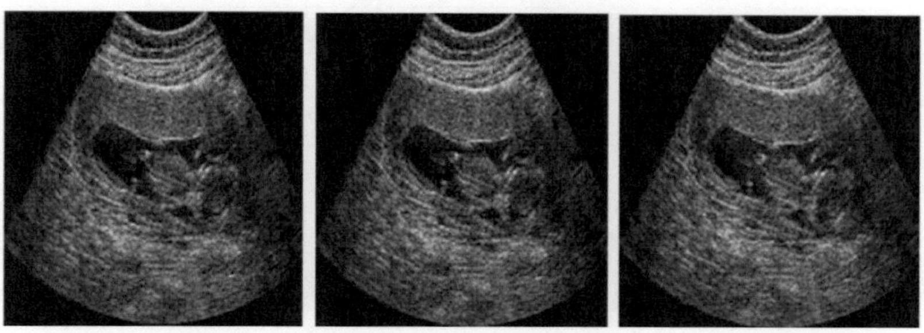

Figure 7. Images from left to right is the synthesized image of placenta obtained from Haar, Daubechies and Symlet Wavelet Decomposition (15 weeks gestational age)

The quality of the image decomposed by different wavelets at various gestational ages is compared in the tables below. The Entropy, Normalized Cross Correlation, Structural Content, Spatial Frequency and Fusion Mutual Information is used as the quality measure in choosing the best wavelet for the characterizing the ultrasound placenta both normal and placenta complicated by GDM. Each has its importance in evaluating the image quality. The entropy of the synthesized image shows an increase in value when, the image is decomposed using Haar Wavelet, compared to the original input images. The measure of structural content of the image is low in the case of Haar. At every level of decomposition, Haar shows good performance in uniquely identifying the features of the placenta. The structural consent is more in the case of Daubechies. The image decomposed using Haar wavelet shows improved quality as the decomposition level increases. In the initial levels, the wavelets, Daubechies, Haar and Symlet show negligible variations in the results. It is also to be noted that placenta with GDM complications are identified by it high entropy when compared to the normal placenta.

The below Table 1 gives the quality evaluation metrics to identify the wavelet, that is suitable for the assessment of ultrasound placenta. Moreover, these metrics shows values with fewer differences between the gestational ages. As the gestational age increases, the metrics also increases.

Wavelet	PSNR	MSE	RMSE	STD	MEAN	Entropy	Class
Haar	33.5101	28.9784	5.3832	43.1958	112.3084	7.4205	Normal
Daubechies	33.4174	29.6035	5.4409	43.054	112.2816	7.3155	
Symlet	33.2889	30.4926	5.522	42.1112	106.5676	7.382	
Haar	33.5476	28.729	5.3599	42.4914	106.5915	7.4491	GDM
Daubechies	34.4057	23.5781	4.8557	42.4914	106.6384	7.3894	
Symlet	33.4628	29.2956	5.4125	44.1209	111.89	7.3894	

The values of PSNR, MSE, RMSE, STD, MEAN, ENTROPY which is recorded in the Table 1, Table 2, Table 3, Table 4 and Table 5 is obtained.

Table 1. Quality Evaluation Metrics to evaluate the performance of Wavelets on normal vs. GDM Ultrasound placenta at 10 weeks of Gestational Age

Wavelet	PSNR	MSE	RMSE	STD	MEAN	Entropy	Class
Haar	33.7862	27.1932	5.2147	63.8662	121.8244	7.4258	Normal
Daubechies	33.6108	28.314	5.3211	63.8403	121.89	7.43	
Symlet	33.5692	28.5864	5.3466	63.803	124.0667	7.4248	
Haar	34.7943	21.5602	4.6433	73.4038	135.7681	7.5319	GDM
Daubechies	34.3782	23.7282	4.8712	73.4146	135.752	7.4496	
Symlet	34.5592	22.7595	4.7707	73.3531	135.7031	7.5122	

Table 2. Quality Evaluation Metrics to evaluate the performance of Wavelets on normal vs. GDM Ultrasound placenta at 12 weeks of Gestational Age

As per the results of the Table 1 and Table 2, the values shows only feeble difference between the normal and the placenta complicated by GDM and also between the Wavelets. At the higher gestational ages as referred in Table 3 and Table 4, there is a distinct demarcation between normal and GDM complication placenta images. Of all these wavelets, Haar shows a remarkable distinction between these features.

The performance of wavelet decomposition of placenta images taken at 15 weeks of gestational Age is shown in Table 3. This gives the metrics that is used to evaluate the normal and GDM Ultrasound placenta.

Wavelet	PSNR	MSE	RMSE	STD	MEAN	Entropy	Class
Haar	34.2999	24.1594	4.9152	34.3881	52.8156	6.5333	Normal
Daubechies	34.0404	25.647	5.0643	34.415	52.9848	6.5404	
Symlet	34.1473	25.0236	5.0024	34.3965	52.7567	6.5357	
Haar	35.6885	17.5481	4.189	32.974	52.3329	6.8749	GDM
Daubechies	35.167	19.7872	4.4483	34.9113	51.5043	6.8435	
Symlet	34.8374	21.3474	4.6203	34.9392	51.4704	6.8632	

The placenta complicated by GDM records higher values when compared to normal. This is clearly indicated in Tables 2, 3, 4 and 5.

Table 3. Quality Evaluation Metrics to evaluate the performance of Wavelets on normal vs. GDM Ultrasound placenta at 15 weeks of Gestational Age

Wavelet	PSNR	MSE	RMSE	STD	MEAN	Entropy	Class
Haar	36.33	15.1383	3.8908	22.5818	45.9544	6.0968	Normal
Daubechies	35.8815	16.7853	4.097	24.6532	55.2264	6.0799	
Symlet	36.115	15.9067	3.9883	24.6608	55.0351	6.0962	
Haar	36.6246	14.1456	3.7611	24.6962	55.074	6.4061	GDM
Daubechies	36.1327	15.8419	3.9802	22.5477	46.0005	6.4017	
Symlet	36.3917	14.9249	3.8633	22.4784	46.2704	6.4053	

Table 4. Quality Evaluation Metrics to evaluate the performance of Wavelets on normal vs. GDM Ultrasound placenta at 17 weeks of Gestational Age

Wavelet	PSNR	MSE	RMSE	STD	MEAN	Entropy	Class
Haar	37.0174	12.9222	3.5948	62.3357	93.3318	6.5345	Normal
Daubechies	35.895	16.7333	4.0906	62.3794	94.6397	6.6267	
Symlet	35.5165	18.2571	4.2728	62.4018	94.7556	6.6428	
Haar	40.2942	6.0766	2.4651	59.9116	94.1953	6.5826	GDM
Daubechies	39.7736	6.8505	2.6173	59.918	94.2794	6.5709	
Symlet	38.8101	8.5521	2.9244	60.005	94.0674	6.6186	

Table 5. Quality Evaluation Metrics to evaluate the performance of Wavelets on normal vs. GDM Ultrasound placenta greater than 20 weeks of Gestational Age

It is clear from the numbers in Table 1 and that the image obtained from Haar Wavelet decomposition performs better than the Daubechies and Symlet decomposition. However, the quality of the input image remains the same irrespective of the decomposition techniques. The high entropy is the indication of the good quality of the image. From the values in Table 6 it can be seen that the wavelet decomposition using Haar dominated the Daubechies and Symlet as indicated by high PSNR of multiview image.

Table 6 suggests that at the higher level of decomposition Haar wavelet gives best results. As the decomposition levels increase the performance of Daubechies and Symlet also increase. It has more or less showed similar results at the first level of decomposition. The entropy of the image considerably increased as the levels improved as in Table 7. At the highest level of decomposition Haar performs better that the other wavelets.

Levels of Decomposition	Haar	Daubechies	Symlet
Level 1	34.4689	33.4174	33.2889
Level 2	36.6246	35.8815	35.6885
Level 3	39.7736	37.0174	36.1357
Level 4	40.3112	39.8702	38.8101

Table 6. PSNR of the different wavelet fused Image at various decomposition levels

Levels of Decomposition	Haar	Daubechies	Symlet
Level 1	6.0799	6.0594	6.0321
Level 2	6.5709	6.4017	6.6267
Level 3	6.6428	6.4674	6.4016
Level 4	7.4491	6.5709	6.5345

Table 7. Entropy of the different wavelet fused Image at various decomposition levels

The results clearly imply that Haar Wavelet yields good quality image at the higher levels of decomposition. The ultrasound images of placenta are then reconstructed using image fusion and it is used to study the complications rendered by GDM on the growth of the placenta.

The low frequency coefficients reflect the approximate feature of the image. It contains the main outline information of the image. It is an approximate image of the original image at certain dimensions. Most of the information and energy of the image is included in this. The high frequency coefficients reflect the detail of the luminance change which corresponds to the edge information of an image. It is important to keep the edge information and the outline information of the input image in the fused image. The fusion should preserve the detail information like high frequency and give prominence to the outline information in the target image. The two images must be of the same size and color map.

3. Wavelet image fusion by max approximation and mean detail

The images decomposed using wavelet techniques are then fused with the original image using min, max and mean fusion techniques. After the fused image is generated, it is processed further and some features of interest are extracted.

In wavelet image fusion scheme, the source images $I_1(x,y)$ and $I_2(x,y)$ are decomposed into approximation and detailed coefficients at required level using Haar Wavelet. The approximation and detailed coefficients of both images are combined using fusion rule. The fused image $I_f(x,y)$ is obtained by taking the inverse wavelet transform. The fusion rule used in this research obtains the maximum of the approximation coefficients and finds the mean of the detailed coefficient in each sub-band with the largest magnitude. Thus using different techniques like mean, max, min approximation and details, fused image is obtained. The inverse 2D wavelet transform is used to reconstruct the image from sub images $I_{LL}(x,y), I_{LH}(x,y), I_{HL}(x,y)$ and $I_{HH}(x,y)$. The Figure 9 show the images fused using the fusion rule (a)Max Max (b) Max Min (c) Max Mean (d) Min Max (e) Min Min (f)Min Mean (g) Mean Max (h) Mean Min (i) Mean Mean approximation and detail of a fetus with the Gestational Age as 15 weeks.

$$I_f(x,y) = fusion\ rule\ \{WT(I_1(x,y)), WT(I_2(x,y))\}$$

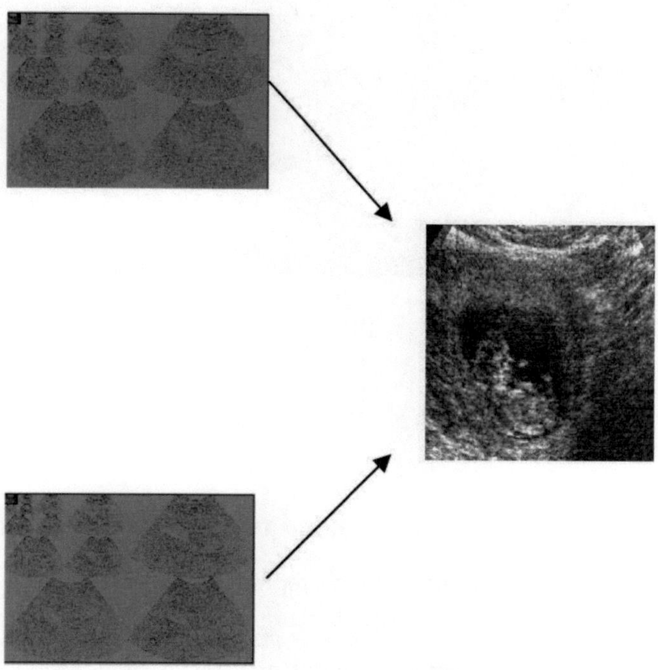

Figure 8. Image Fusion of Wavelet Decomposed Ultrasound Placenta using Max Approximation and Mean Detail

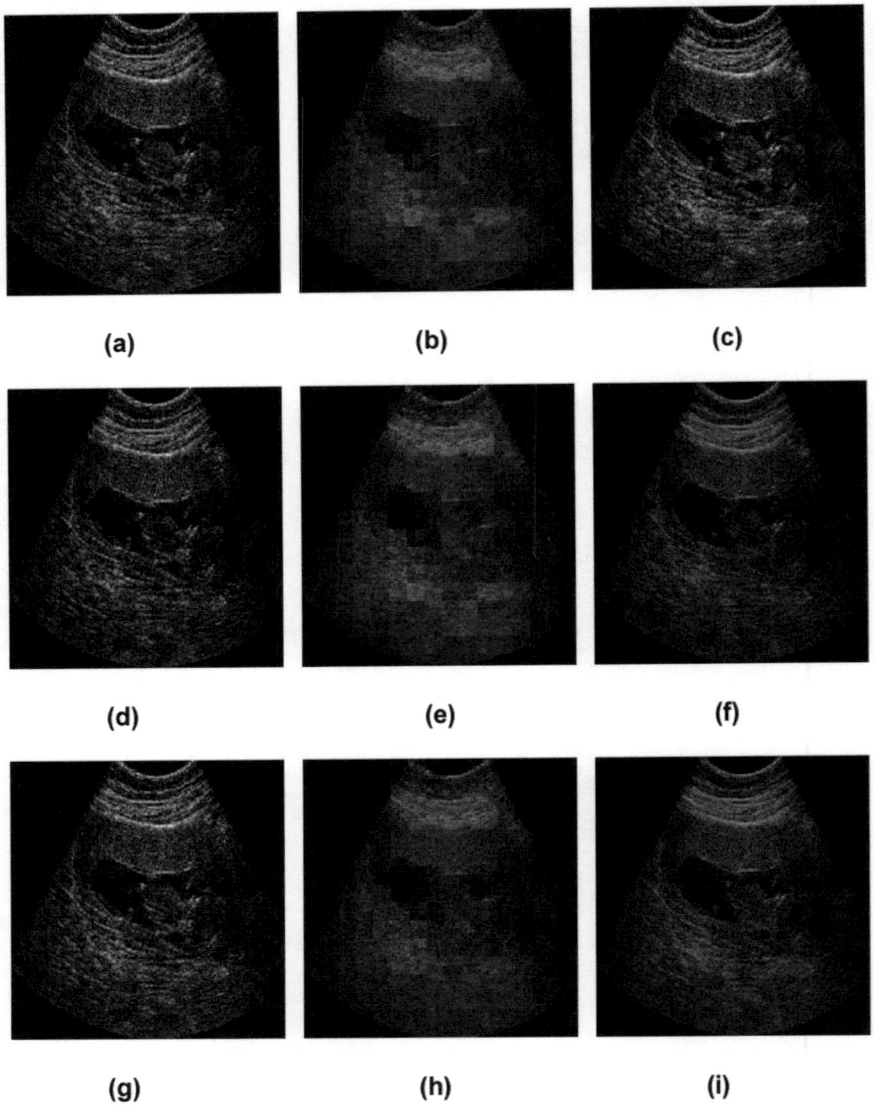

Figure 9. Image fused using the fusion rule (a) Max Max (b) Max Min (c) Max Mean (d) Min Max (e) Min Min (f)Min Mean (g) Mean Max (h) Mean Min (i) Mean Mean approximation and detail of 15 weeks of Gestational Age

4. Diagnostic accuracy evaluation of fused ultrasound placenta

In the case of medical images, it is important to reproduce the image close to the original image so that the smallest of the details are readable.

This research used image quality measures like Entropy, Mean, Standard Deviation, Fusion Mutual Information, Normalized Cross Correlation, Root Mean Square Error, Structural content, Normalized Absolute Error and Absolute Difference to analyze on the fused image.

Though the fusion methods produced varieties of images, few fusion rules only produced images suitable for diagnostic accuracy. A useful image is identified on the execution of quality measures on these images. The quality measures obtained for the images fused with different fusion rules is recorded in Table 8and Table 9. The values for PSNR, RMSE, NAE, NCC, SC, FMI, ENT, MEAN, STD and AD recorded in Tables 8 and 9 are obtained. The PSNR value obtained for Max Mean Fusion Rule performed well compared to other fusion rule followed by Min Mean. The recording to the table 8 and 9 shows Max Mean with lower RMSE value indicating the closeness of the fused image to the original image. Similar is the NAE results. The quality measure NCC shows good performance of Mean Max followed by Max Max. The structural Content ranks Max Max as good fusion rule followed by Max Min, Min Mean and then Max Mean. The values depicted in Tables 8 and 9 shows that Max Mean as the best quality image which shows high FMI and Entropy. These indicate the richness of information. The Mean and STD play only a less role in the selection of fusion rule for the fused ultrasound placenta image. Again AD shows Max Mean fused image to be cleaner that the other rules. It clearly shows that the wavelet decomposed images when subjected to image fusion increases the quality of information in an image. Thus the essential features, that characterizes the placenta can extracted. It preserves boundary information and structural details without introducing any other consistencies to the image. This work suggests that Max Approximation and Mean Detail fusion rule produces good quality ultrasound placenta complicated by GDM followed by Max Approximation and Max Detail fusion rule.

Fusion Rule		PSNR	RMSE	NAE	NCC	SC
Approximation	**Detail**					
Max	Max	38.2766	3.1096	0.121	1.008	0.9548
Max	Min	39.5058	2.6993	0.0893	1.0065	0.9702
Max	**Mean**	40.9709	2.2803	0.0637	1.0066	0.9782
Min	Max	39.3109	2.7605	0.0951	0.9941	0.9923
Min	Min	39.7844	2.6141	0.0819	0.991	1.0023
Min	Mean	40.5563	2.3918	0.071	0.9914	1.0062
Mean	Max	38.9197	2.8877	0.1013	1.0083	0.9616
Mean	Min	39.5153	2.6964	0.089	0.9991	0.9842
Mean	Mean	40.253	2.4768	0.0747	1.0052	0.9774

Table 8. Evaluation of fusion rules based on Image Quality Measures PSNR, RMSE, NAE, NCC and SC

The pelvic ultrasound image taken during the first and second trimester of pregnancy shows the fetus, placenta and the cervix. It is essential to segment the region of interest, which is the placenta, from the ultrasound. The wavelet decomposed placenta ultrasound is segmented to extract the area of focus, placenta. The statistical measures to estimate the volume of the placenta, are obtained from this segmented placenta ultrasound. The relevant image features are then extracted from the segmented placenta. Neural Network is an efficient tool that can capture and represent complex input and output relationship. The reconstructed placenta ultrasound is later classified as either normal placenta or abnormal placenta, using the extracted features.

Fusion Rule		FMI	ENT	MEAN	STD	AD
Approximation	**Detail**					
Max	Max	38.2766	3.1096	0.121	1.008	-0.5526
Max	Min	39.5058	2.6993	0.0893	1.0065	-0.4963
Max	**Mean**	40.9709	2.2803	0.0637	1.0066	-0.8875
Min	Max	39.3109	2.7605	0.0951	0.9941	0.0208
Min	Min	39.7844	2.6141	0.0819	0.991	-0.3151
Min	Mean	40.5563	2.3918	0.071	0.9914	0.0022
Mean	Max	38.9197	2.8877	0.1013	1.0083	-0.4466

Table 9. Evaluation of fusion rules based on Image Quality Measures FMI, ENT, MEAN and STD

The present research also evaluates the influence of GDM on adverse outcomes of pregnancy by an estimation of volume of the placenta during the early stages of pregnancy. During the course of pregnancy, ultrasound screenings are done in early pregnancy which is from six to fourteen weeks of gestation. The mid pregnancy is from fourteen to twenty six weeks of gestation. The late pregnancy is from twenty six to forty weeks of gestation. In the later stages of gestation, the fetus in the uterus hides the placenta and therefore makes it difficult to get it captured in the ultrasound. The focus of this research is the ultrasound placenta with 10 weeks, 15 weeks, 17 weeks and more than 20 weeks as the gestational age. The placenta needs to be screened in the initial stages, which can avoid miscarriages due to GDM. The standard common obstetric diagnostic mode is 2D scanning. The estimation of placental volume is not a regular practice in the case of 2D ultrasound. The results of the work have effectively identified the changes in the ultrasound placenta under diabetic conditions.

The findings of the research are that the Haralick features extraction showed significant characteristics of abnormal placenta. Energy, entropy, contrast, homogeneity and correlation features are often used among the 14 Haralick texture features to reveal certain properties about the spatial distribution of the texture image. Since real textures usually have so many different dimensions, these texture properties are not independent of each other. For instance, the energy measure generated from gray level co-occurrence matrix is also known as homogeneity and variance is a measure of contrast in images. Therefore, when choosing a subset of meaningful features from gray level co-occurrence matrix for a particular application, features do not have to be independent because a subset of fully independent features is usually hard to find. These features played an important role in the identification of abnormal placenta. It is found that there is an increase in classification accuracy when placenta ultrasound is subjected to wavelet decomposition and image fusion.

The Haralick features which are obtained from the ultrasound images are recorded in the following Table 10. This table shows the discriminating features that aid in the classification of normal placenta and placenta complicated by gestational diabetes mellitus. The features Mean, Contrast, Correlation, Entropy recorded in the Table 10

Images	Mean	Contrast	Correlation	Entropy	Sum of squares	Class
Img1	1.635 e4	1310473767	7.922339e5	8.944150e4	7.2	AN
Img2	1.832 e4	1614852030	2.978678e6	1.047565e5	1.1	AN
Img3	1.454 e4	1434646325	1.911394e5	9.609855e4	5.6	AN(GDM)
Img4	1.455 e4	1436691775	1.915322e5	9.670916e4	1.0	AN
Img5	1.222 e4	1077321331	1.055089e5	7.347292e4	1.2	N
Img6	1.832 e4	1614852030	2.978678e6	1.047565e5	2.5	AN
Img7	1.854 e4	1647605895	9.059511e5	7.575653e4	1.7	AN
Img8	1.749 e4	1531849951	7.756140e5	9.824614e4	2.15	AN
Img9	1.263 e4	1083142018	1.065980e5	7.3943192e4	1.2	N
Img10	1.280 e4	1067278301	1.059341e5	7.367722e4	1.14	N

Table 10. Haralick Features for Ultrasound Placenta Images for sample images

The Haralick features that were extracted from the wavelet fused ultrasound placenta, highlights on the characteristic features of the input image. These features form the basis for effective classification of placenta whether it is normal or complicated by gestational diabetes mellitus.

Image segmentation refers to the process of partitioning of an image into groups of pixels which are homogeneous with respect to some criterion. Segmentation algorithms have a limited application in ultrasound image. The presence of high levels of speckling in ultrasound images makes accurate segmentation difficult. The region of interest is typically obtained through manual interaction. The original gray-scale image is first converted to binary image using optimal global image threshold. Next the image complement is defined. Image transform using the watershed method should be applied to a matrix after its proper preprocessing to obtain the best image objects contours. The segmented image is obtained using the watershed segmentation method. It starts with a pixel or a group of pixels called seeds that belong to the structure of interest. Seeds are chosen by the operator.

The watershed segmentation algorithm is applied on the synthesized placenta image which gives the segmentation of the placenta from the ultrasound as given in the Figure 10 below.

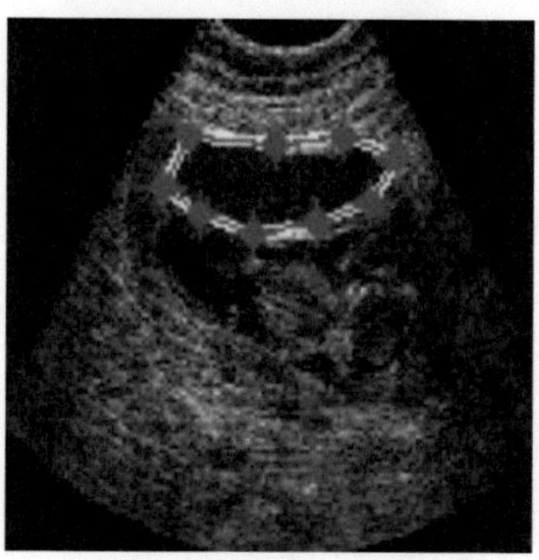

Figure 10. Watershed Segmentation of Ultrasound Placenta

The contour is traced for the segmented placenta which is marked in the Figure 10 as dotted lines. The contour extracted ultrasound placenta is displayed below.

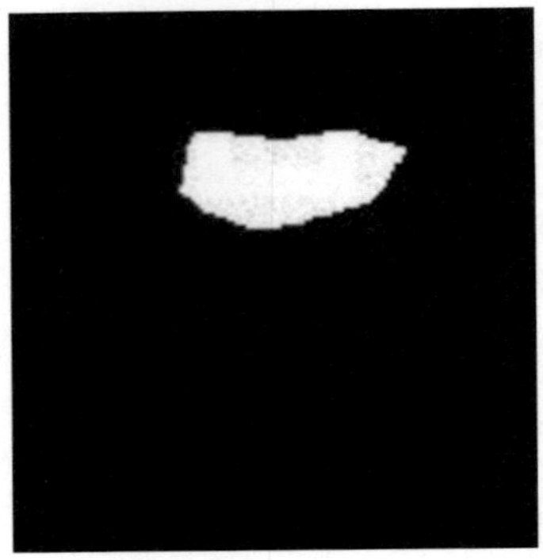

Figure 11. Contour Extracted Ultrasound Placenta

The segmented binary image of the placenta is displayed in the Figure 12 which is used to generate the parameters required for volume estimation.

5. Statistical measurement of segmented region

The statistical measures often give characteristic parameters on the interested image. There is a need for the measurement of major axis length. The complications in placenta that occur during pregnancy show some variations in the size of the placenta. There arise the need for the measurement of major axis length and minor axis length of the segmented placenta. With these statistical values one can obtain the area and perimeter of the segmented image. These values are then recorded to delineate the normal placenta and the placenta complicated by gestational diabetes mellitus. The distance measure tool is used to obtain the thickness of the placenta.

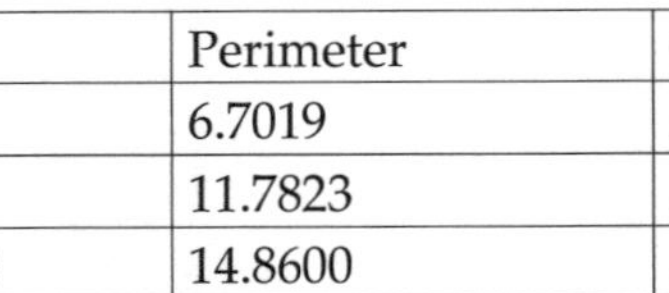

Figure 12. Segmented Binary Image of Ultrasound Placenta

Images	Area	Perimeter	Class
Image1	3.2167	6.7019	AN
Image2	6.0015	11.7823	AN
Image3	10.2083	14.8600	AN (GDM)
Image4	6.8913	9.9025	AN
Image5	7.3428	10.3109	N

Table 11. Statistical Measurement of Area, Perimeter of the Segmented Ultrasound Placenta

The limitation in the ultrasound scanning prevents monitoring the growth of the placenta. Placental volume assessment is uncommon in routine obstetric practice, a lack that prevents obstetricians from identifying their patients with extremely small or large placentas.

6. Convex concave shell model

A new method to determine the volume of the two dimensional ultrasound placentas using a mathematical model is proposed. The aim of the work is to correlate the height, width and thickness of the ultrasound placenta in measuring the placental volume.

The shape of the placenta in general is a round or oval. Using this as reference, the major axis length (l) and minor axis length (b) of the ultrasound placenta of a segmented image is obtained using *'regionprops'* in Matlab 7.0. The thickness (h) of the placenta was obtained from the point of chord insertion. This was obtained using the measure tool in Matlab 7.0. The mathematical representation of the segmented placenta is shown in Figure 13. The feasibility for classifying the ultrasound images of placenta with complicating diabetes based on placenta thickness using statistical textural features was analyzed.

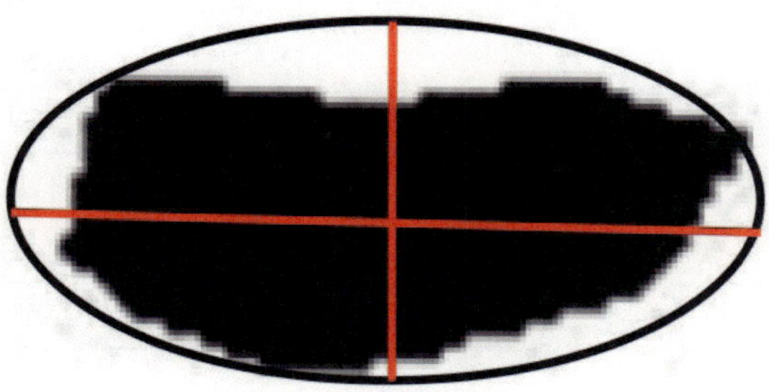

Figure 13. Measurement of Major Axis Length and Minor Axis Length to calculate Area and Perimeter

The concave-convex shell formula

$$V = \left(\left(\frac{\pi h}{6}\right) * [4b(l-h) + l(l-4h) + 4h^2]\right) \quad (1)$$

Where,

h=Thickness, b=Minor Axis Length, l=Major Axis Length

The high values of major axis length and minor axis length strongly indicate placenta complicated by gestational diabetes mellitus.

The Figure 14 represents the mathematical model of volume estimation from the ultrasound images of placenta. The volume estimated by measuring the length (black marker) of the placenta, height of the placenta (green marker) as seen in ultrasound and the thickness (red marker) measured from point of chord insertion.

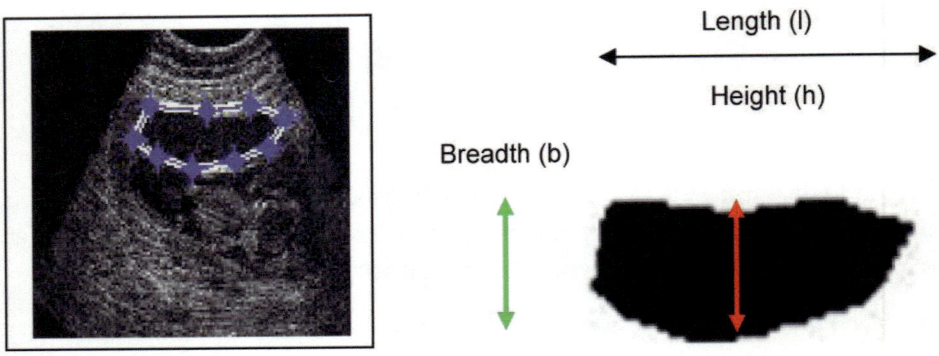

Figure 14. Concave-Convex Shell Representation of Ultrasound Placenta

Img Id	Major Axis Length (l)	Minor Axis Length (b)	Height (h)	Volume (V)	Class
Img1	7.482	3.79	2.31	104.689004	1
Img2	13.72	4.63	3.6	433.1933952	2
Img3	5.76	4.13	0.98	47.90461872	0
Img4	7.9	3.71	1.54	94.78968781	1
Img5	6.95	3.51	1.9	80.3664945	1
Img6	7.482	3.79	2.31	104.689004	1
Img7	14.78	4.01	4.78	469.4087275	2
Img8	5.23	2.1	1.98	29.95954698	0

Table 12. Volume Estimation from Statistical Parameters

7. Conclusion

The study concludes that the application of wavelet decomposition reduces the speckle in the ultrasound placenta. The fusion of such decomposed wavelet improves the characteristics of the essential features which in turn, enhances the classification accuracy. The Haralick features obtained for the ultrasound image of placenta plays a significant role in the classification process. There is also an increase in the contrast of ultrasound placenta which is complicated by GDM. The outcome of the research is that, multi-view scans can be fused to identify the influence of GDM on the early stage of placental growth by employing wavelet decomposition and image fusion technique. This research also suggests that, the evaluation of the volume of placenta during the routine ultrasound screening at fifteen to twenty weeks of gestation using wavelet fusion of multi-view of the ultrasound placenta can identify the influence of diabetes mellitus which otherwise can lead to the severe risk of fetal demise.

Author details

G. Malathi
*School of Computer Science and Engineering, VIT University-Chennai Campus
Chennai, India*

V. Shanthi
*Department of MCA, St. Joseph's College of Engineering, Affiliated to Anna University,
Chennai, India*

8. References

[1] http://en.wikipedia.org/wiki/Placenta (Archived from the original on 6 January 2008)

[2] Sicree R. Shaw J. Zimmet P. Diabetes and impaired glucose tolerance. In: Diabetes Atlas. International Diabetes Federation.(ed). Belgium: International Diabetes Federation; 2006. p.15-103.

[3] http://en.wikipedia.org/wiki/Computer-aided_diagnosis (Accessed 12 September 2009).

[4] India has largest number of diabetes patients – Report. www.indianexpress.com/news/india-has-largest-number-of-diabetes-patient /531240/ (Accessed 21 October 2009).

[5] www.fortishospitals.com/associate-specialities/

[6] diabetology_and_endocrinology.html (Accessed 10 February 2011)

[7] Muhammad Ashfaq, Muhammad ZahoorJanjua, Muhammad Aslam Channa. Effect of gestational diabetes and maternal hypertension on gross morphology of placenta. Journal of Ayub Medical College; http://www.ayubmed.edu.pk/JAMC/PAST/17-1/Ashfaq.htm (Accessed 13 October 2011)

[8] Metzger BE, Coustan DR(Eds). Gestational Diabetes Mellitus. Diabetes Care: 4th International Workshop – Conference Proceedings. Vol. 21(Suppl. 2). p. B1-B167; 1998.

[9] Gestational Diabetes Mellitus. American Diabetes Association, Diabetes Care. vol. 27. p. 88-90; 2004.

[10] Seshiah V. Prevalence of Gestational Diabetes Mellitus in South India (Tamil Nadu) – A Community Based Study. JAPI. vol.56; 2008.

[11] EberhardMerz F. Bahlmann. Ultrasound in Obstetrics and Gynecology. vol.1. Thieme; 2005.

[12] http://www.pregnancycheck.com/pregnancy-ultrasound.html (Accessed 29 August 2011).

[13] JosipDjelmis. GernotDesoye. Marina Ivanisevic. Diabetology of pregnancy: Karger.

[14] Novel study in TN to know gestational diabetes effects. The Hindu. Health – Medicine & Research. (Accessed on 8 March 2012).

[15] BhanuPrakash K.N. et al. Lung Maturity Analysis Using Ultrasound Image Features. IEEE Transactions on Information Technology in Biomedicine 2002;6(1) 38-45.

[16] Thomose R. Moore et al. Diabetes Mellitus and Pregnancy. eMedicine. http://emedicine.medscape.com/article/127547-overview (Accessed 3 February 2012)
[17] www.pregnancy-info.net/placental_abruption.html (Accessed 23 May 2010)

Chapter 6

Periodontitis and Diabetes Mellitus

Michal Straka and Michaela Straka-Trapezanlidis

Additional information is available at the end of the chapter

http://dx doi.org/10.5772/50269

1. Introduction

Diabetes mellitus is a serious metabolic disease and an important medical, social and economic problem globally. Long-term untreated hyperglycaemia – the main cause of a carbohydrate, lipid and osmotic imbalance – affects all tissues and organs in the body and leads to development of typical disease manifestations such as polydipsia, polyuria and polyphagia. This metabolic imbalance initiates other tissue and organ complications, some of which are extremely serious vasculopathies, cardiovascular diseases, neuropathies, myopathies, eye complications, renal complications and deteriorated regeneration and healing of wounds (Ceriello, 2005).

The basic etiopathogenetic mechanism in diabetes mellitus is either a real lack of insulin (type 1) or a biological lack of insulin (type 2) arising from its peripherally changed utilization and subsequent insufficiency. Insulin is a polypeptide produced by beta-cells of the pancreas and is necessary for glucose metabolism, keeping the glucose level in the blood within values of 4 – 6 mmol/1 ml. Glucose is metabolized in all tissues and is the main energy source in the organism. Lack of insulin causes hyperglycaemia and unmetabolised glucose is excreted mostly by the kidneys. This state leads to the development of polyuria, requiring increased intake of liquids and food and causing tissues to metabolise other sources of energy (fats, proteins) much more. Insufficient effectiveness of insulin means the energy requirements of the organism are not fulfilled; the organism searches for additional energy sources, mainly for proteins and fats. Increased metabolism of fats leads to excretion of so-called keto-compounds by the kidneys accompanied by a typical smell which can be detected in the patient's breath and sweat.

Nowadays we divide diabetes mellitus into the insulin-dependent type 1 DM, also called children's or adolescent DM, which presents an absolute lack of insulin caused by the autoimmune destruction of pancreatic beta-cells; and type 2 DM, which is known as adult diabetes, is a more frequent form of this illness and runs without clinical symptoms for a longer time. The initial stages of the disease are characterized by insulin-tissue resistance connected with inadequate glucose tolerance. Increased insulin resistance of receptors and tissue produces an increased insulin requirement and forces its production in the pancreas. If insulin production in the pancreas drops below 50 per cent, a so-called pre-diabetic condition develops. This is characterized by after-strain hyperglycaemia, also called postprandial hyperglycaemia, which often runs sub-clinically. If it remains undiagnosed, it can develop into a more advanced form with various tissue and organ complications, oral manifestations and complications (Straka, 2011). The most frequent oral complications of diabetes are diabetes gingivitis and periodontitis, which are together considered to be the seventh most common complication of DM. In type 2 diabetes, the incidence of periodontitis is 2.9 – 3.0 times higher than in non-diabetic patients (Nelson et al., 1990; Tsai et al., 2002).

2. Classification of diabetes mellitus

The present classification of diabetes mellitus uses the AAD (American Association of Diabetes) division and distinguishes four types of DM.

1. Type 1 DM – autoimmune type (older synonym is IDDM – insulin-dependent diabetes mellitus), diabetes of young people;
2. Type 2 DM – non-autoimmune (an older synonym is NIDDM – non-insulin-dependent diabetes mellitus), diabetes of adults, insulin non-resistant type;
3. Specific types of DM
4. Gestational DM (Straka, 2001; Farkaš et al., 2011).

3. Etiopathogenesis of DM and diabetic periodontitis

3.1. Type 1 diabetes mellitus (T1DM)

T1DM starts as an autoimmune and destructive reaction against the patient's own pancreatic beta-cells. The main risk factor is a genetic predisposition to such an autoimmune reaction. Some authors distinguish six stages of T1DM development described as follows: the 1st stage, known as genetic predisposition, passes into the 2nd so-called activating stage, which is characterized by immediate activation of autoimmune reactions. The 3rd stage, for which immune abnormalities are typical, passes into the 4th stage characterized by loss of glucose-stimulating insulin production. Clinically present diabetes in the 5th stage is a reflection of the large destruction of B-cells and leads to their total destruction in the 6th and final stage (Rybka, 1990). In young patients with T1DM, an increased susceptibility to gingivitis and periodontitis has been detected. This state is often accompanied by more extensive damage to periodontal tissue and an early onset of gingivitis after the patients reach the age of 11. Periodontal pockets were detected in 9.8% of a group of young patients aged 13 – 18 years, compared with a 1.7% occurrence in a healthy control group (Straka, 2001; Rybka, 1990).

3.1.1. *Etiopathogenic and risk factors*

An increased prevalence of gingivitis and periodontitis in adolescents with T1DM is mostly attributed to various etiopathogenetic and risk factors of the primary illness:

Altered immunity. The most frequent immunological disorder is an excessive production of the pro-inflammatory cytokines TNF-alpha, IL-1, PGE2 and others. They induce hyper-inflammatory systemic or local status and contribute to chronicity due to prolonged inflammation. The immune system is unable to eliminate significantly gram-negative bacteria from the subgingival area. The causes can be genetically determined in a form of dangerous phenotype of monocytes/macrophages and their increased inflammatory reaction to the LPS toxin as well as various polymorphisms of inflammatory mediators (Straka, 2001; Salvi et al. 1997).

Tissue glycation. Long-lasting hyperglycaemia initiates the rise of so-called non-enzymatic tissue glycosylation, which causes formation of AGEs (Advanced Glycosylation End-products). Increased amounts of AGEs condition a growth of receptors and cause all attendant changes in vascular structures and increased formation of inflammatory cytokines, adhesive molecules and other immunocompetent substances with possible subsequent multiplication of bacterial pathogens (Gislen et al., 1980; Mealey & Oates, 2006; Mandell et al, 1992).

Disorders of tissue regeneration and wound healing. Tissue glycation and expansion of inflammation in T1DM patients seem to be a cause of deterioration in the regenerative abilities of periodontal tissue, including osseous structures, which are measured by means of bone-building biomarkers such as osteocalcin, the values of which were reduced in comparison with the control group of non-diabetic patients (Lappin et al., 2009).

3.1.2. *Influence of T1DM treatment on the state and course of periodontitis*

Several studies report that balanced levels of glycaemia in T1DM patients have a beneficial influence on the degree of periodontal tissue damage during periodontitis as well as on its clinical course. These results associate total systemic changes with destructive changes to the periodontium depending on the therapeutic result of the glycaemia level. The given relationship acts reciprocally. (Straka, 2001; Farkaš et al., 2011; Cianciola et al. 1982, Lyons, 1992) However the results of other present-day clinical studies negate the positive correlation between periodontal therapy and its beneficial influence on the course of the primary illness. Periodontal therapy in T1DM subjects prevented periodontal infection, but did not significantly influence the level of glycated haemoglobin (Tervonen et al., 2009). Statistically insignificant results of periodontological therapy on glycated haemoglobin concentrations have also been confirmed by another independent study (Lambés et al., 2008).

3.2. Type 2 diabetes mellitus (T2DM)

The etiopathogenesis of T2DM and its most frequent oral complication are closely interconnected. Their mutual associations can be observed in various stages of the primary disease. One of the early pathological symptoms of broken homeostasis of glucose is its increased postprandial (after-strain) level in the blood. This type of hyperglycaemia is bound to food and develops several years before it is clinically manifested by T2DM. The pre-diabetic stage of the disease is characterized by the presence of several markers, of which the most important is glycated haemoglobin A1c, which represents the amount of glycated haemoglobin in erythrocytes (given in percentages). The pre-diabetic stage of the disease, measured by means of HB1c, FPG, and 2-hOGTT can be relevant in the development of some angiopathies, mainly retinopathy (Ceriello, 2005; Straka, 2011; Rybka, 1990). In T2DM aetiology as well as in the development of diabetic periodontitis, the following groups of factors and mechanisms play crucial roles:

Genetic associations. For some multifactoral diseases several genes were selected using relevant literature gene databases and listed by statistic methods into individual groups according to their severity. The most important group is formed by so-called leader genes, characteristic for both diseases (Covani et al. 2008). After their application into the databases of two leader genes selected from 986 genes for T2DM, four leader genes actively acting in both diseases were identified. The most significant of them was NFKB1, whose increased activity was detected in periodontal lesions and which seems to have a relationship with microvascular defects induced by a systemic inflammatory process. Another leader gene is RELA, which together with NFKB1 codes two subunits of the complex NFKB triggering an intracellular inflammatory reaction (Covani, Marconcini, Derchi; 2009). STRING software enabled us to determine a close association between periodontitis and T2DM by means of IL-6 and TNF-alpha (Covani et al., (2009); Nishimuraet al., 2003). It is also true that there are certain limitations in the given theoretical knowledge and that by removing these limitations, scientific research could more strongly validate the presented knowledge (Covani et al., 2009). Nowadays our ability to determine dangerous genetic predispositions to T2DM by means of certain genetic profiles, in wide populations, remains considerably limited. Genetic risk factors certainly play an important role in the etiopathogenesis of T2DM, genome-wide association studies having stated that genetic RF can be useful in establishing certain profiles of disease susceptibility and can be used in T2DM disease and therapy management (Khoury et al., 2008).

Insulin resistance. In type 2 diabetes mellitus, there is sufficient insulin at an early stage of the disease, a fact confirmed by an abundance of B-cells in pancreatic tissues. But their effectiveness in producing insulin varies and is influenced by the progress of the disease, level of abdominal obesity and other factors. At the beginning of the disease there is enough insulin, but relevant structures are metabolically so altered that biological utilization of insulin is insufficient. Insulin in tissues and cells acts by means of its receptors, which are of glycoprotein character. A starting signal of cellular activity of insulin is activation by receptor tyrosine kinases, which phosphorylate substrates of insulin receptors in tyrosine residues. Glucose transport is ensured by a lipid kinase and is stimulated by P13K into its fully active form determined for glucose transport by means of insulin. However these mechanisms are extremely complicated and there are several possible ways this complicated mechanism of glucose may function. The relationship between insulin and lipogenesis as well as the effects of various transcription factors in adipocyte are also very complicated (Nishimura et. al., 2003; Kahn & Flier, 2000). Both the prevalence and etiopathogenesis of T2DM are nowadays most often associated with obesity, mainly of the abdominal type. "Insulin resistance" is not an insulin-induced disorder of glucose metabolism, but an expression of decreased insulin-induced transport of glucose and its metabolism in striated muscles and adipocytes (Nishimura et al., 2003; Kahn & Flier, 2000; Watanabe et al., 2008; Al-Zahrani et al., 2003). Insulin controls glucose homeostasis in the blood, decreasing its level by reduced production in liver and increased absorption in muscles and adipose tissues. The most frequent disorders of insulin activity are defects of its signal systems, mainly in the adipocytes. These require higher effort to get insulin and to produce it in larger amounts, which leads to hyperinsulinemia. Excess levels of insulin in the blood can result in a receptors imbalance and loss of post-receptor sensitivity; all this can be accompanied by glucose intolerance and age-related insufficiency of insulin receptors (Kahn & Flier, 2000). Increased serum concentrations of fatty acids (usually connected with diabetes and T2DM) contribute to further development of insulin resistance. Excessive levels of fatty acids in blood and muscles brake phosphorylation and transport of glucose as well as the synthesis of muscular glycogen and subsequent glucose oxidation (Kahn & Flier, 2000; Ferenčík & Hulín, 2008; Shulman, 2000).

Metabolic syndrome. Obesity, hyperlipidaemia and insulin resistance are the principal symptoms of metabolic syndrome. Obesity also leads to other factors that contribute to metabolic syndrome. One of the dominant factors is dyslipidaemia characterized by increased triglyceride concentration, non-esterified fatty acids as well as a higher concentration of specific LDLs, also called low-density lipoprotein particles. Dyslipidaemia is accompanied by low HDL cholesterol levels. Nowadays it is obvious that individual components of metabolic syndrome represent independent risk factors in the etiopathogenesis of insulin resistance. Their mutual communicative effect also exists (Ferenčík & Hulín, 2008; Shulman, 2000; Coenen et al., 2007). Adipose tissue in obese people has various forms. As for formation of pro-inflammatory cytokines, the most harmful is white adipose tissue in the abdominal region, which contains residual macrophages (Straka, 2011; Coenen et al., 2007). Formation of inflammatory cytokines in these macrophages significantly increases the pro-inflammatory status of the organism with all its consequences. Adipocytes are the principal cells of adipose tissues and are excreted with the endocrine function. One of the most important products is leptin characterized by its pleiotropic effect, which plays an important role in energy-balance regulation. Adipocytes produce substances which have either a direct or indirect relation to insulin resistance. Production of pro-inflammatory cytokines and TNF-alpha, IL-6, CRP markers, angiotensinogen, but also of steroid hormones of oestrogen and cortisol, contribute to local biology of adipose tissue. Increased production of TNF-alpha increases lipolysis and inhibits lipogenesis, which together with other co-factors, leads to insulin resistance (Ferenčík & Hulín, 2008; Shulman, 2000; Coenen et al., 2007).

Inflammation and insulin resistance. Type 2 diabetes, insulin resistance and obesity with dyslepidaemia are pro-inflammatory states which are closely interconnected. While leptin and adiponektin are exclusively products of adipocytes, TNF-alpha, IL-6, MCP-1, resistin, visfatin and PAI-1 are produced by activated macrophages and other cells, and contribute to the maintenance and stimulation of low-grade inflammation in obesity (Straka, 2011; Shoelson, Jongsoon, Goldifine, 2006). The inflammatory kinases JNK, IKKbeta, PKC, STAT cause insulin resistance by decreasing insulin signalization on receptors (Kim et al., 2004; Mehta et al., 2010). Nowadays inflammatory cytokines, mainly TNF-alpha, represent important etiopathogenic factors of insulin resistance stimulation. Together with the LPS-toxin of periodontal bacterial pathogens, they activate NF-kapaB, which after displacement into the cell nuclei can induce insulin resistance (Ceriello, 2005; Salvi et al. 1997). Patients with the abdominal type of obesity show increased TNF-alpha serum levels, which drop with decrease of body mass (Gislen et al., 1980). Increased TNF-alpha levels and other pro-inflammatory mediators circulating in patients with metabolic syndrome can stimulate inflammation of the periodontium, where also in clinically healthy individuals, gram-negative anaerobic bacteria are present, and induce increased proteolytic and osteolytic destruction of tissues (Salvi et al., 1997; Mealey & Oates, 2006). Increased prevalence of periodontal illnesses in the obese, mainly in younger individuals, has also been confirmed by a NHANES III study involving 13,655 patients, who were tested according to periodontal indices (PD, AL) and BMI and WC indices. A correlation between these two diseases was established by using two different multivariable logistic regressive models containing other risk factors in periodontal disorders (sex, race, education, diabetes, smoking habits, date of last visit to the dentist) (Mandell et al., 1992). Nowadays the secreting activity of the adipocytes of adipose tissues is considered a source of chronic low-grade inflammation as well as an important pro-inflammatory etiopathogenetic factor in many serious diseases, including type 2 diabetes and inflammatory-destructive illnesses of the periodontium (Ceriello, 2005; Lappin, et al., 2009; Lyons, 1992).

Non-enzymatic glycation. Non-enzymatic glycation presents a basic chemical reaction by which glucose is bound to lysine residues and, by means of unstable or stable intermediate products, forms so-called advanced glycosylation end products. Production and accumulation of AGEs runs also in periodontal tissues and has an influence on their composition and immunological qualities in several possible ways. In a normal glycaemic regime AGE-receptors are present in small amounts in monocytes, smooth muscle cells, neurons, fibroblasts and endothelial cells. Increased levels of AGE-receptors can lead to overproduction of adhesive molecules and oxidative elements, the consequence of which is an increased uncontrolled anti-inflammatory immune response to the presence of microbial pathogens in the periodontium (Tervonen et al., 2009). Another serious factor in a severe anti-inflammatory reaction is excessive activity of proteolytic enzymes, which destroy periodontal soft tissues. Several studies have confirmed an increased concentration of metalloproteinases in the periodontium of a diabetic patient. These are caused by increased transcription of local resident cells stimulated by overproduction of pro-inflammatory cytokines (Lambés et al. (2008). Collagen glycation results in strengthening of cross-links among its molecules, impairing solubility, natural homeostasis and biological regenerative qualities. Regeneration of ageing collagen and basal membrane is reduced and accumulation of AGEs products in these structures starts (Covani et al., (2008). Destruction of the periodontium correlates with imbalanced glycaemic curve as well as with a level of glycated haemoglobin. In diabetic patients with an HbA1c level higher than 8 %, their IL-1beta concentration was found to be two times higher than in patients with an HbA1c level lower than 8 % (Covani et al., 2009). The level of glycaemic control and length of diabetic disease have an impact on the stage of glycation and collagen regeneration in soft and osseous tissues. Defects in osteoblast differentiation and altered production of extracellular matrix contribute to this state (Cianciola et al., 1982; Nishimura et al., 2003). On the basis of given studies we can conclude that the glycation of various components of periodontal tissues significantly changes its immunity to various exogene elements (bacteria, viruses) and considerably decreases regeneration and healing of these tissues.

Defects in cell-mediated immunity. In subjects with DM, defects of polymorphonuclear leukocytes have been repeatedly confirmed. These are based in defects of chemotaxis and phagocytosis and result in insufficient antibacterial protection of periodontal structures (McMullen et al., 1981; King, 2008). In subjects with DM, the hypersecretive type of monocytes was detected, which on irritation with LPS-endotoxin gram-negative periodontopathic bacteria reacted with increased IL-lbeta and TNF-alpha production, which stimulated inflammation of periodontal tissues with excessively destructive osteolysis and tissue destruction of periodontal ligaments (Collins et al., 1997; Galbraith et al., 1998).

Influence of microbial factors. Altered immunity, vasculopathy of periodontal structures, decreased solubility of glycated tissues, defects of protein and osseous regeneration and repair all cause that immunity of the periodontium to typical periodontal pathogens is considerably reduced and is less effective against infections. Some studies report differences between groups of patients with long-lasting and correctly managed monitoring of glycaemia and those with an insufficiently monitored and managed course of glycaemia. Increased amounts of periodontal microbial pathogens were confirmed in diabetic patients but their microbial strains were no different from those of non-diabetic patients (Mandel et al. 1992; Zambon et al., 1988; Straka, 2011).

3.3. Gestational DM (GDM)

Gestational DM is characterized with high blood sugar levels inpregnant women, who were not diagnosed for DM previously. Its prevalencein pregnant women varies from 5 to 7 percent. Usually is concern atransient form, while placental and maternal adipose tissues producehormones which can change metabolism of glucose (Friedlander et al.,2007). Some authors state that in up to 50 per cent of women with GDM,T2DM can develop within 3.5 years. Although there is lack of relevantstudies to this topic and no anonymous conclusion was done, most authorsconfirm the hypothesis that pregnant women with GDM have a high risk todevelop a severe form of an inflammatory diseases of the periodont (Novak et al.,2006; Friedlander et al., 2007; Xiong, et al., 2006). Thisrelationship runs in both directions and presence of inflammatorydiseases unfavorably influences the mother's organism and the healthstate of the foetus (Novak et al., 2006; Straka et al., 2011).

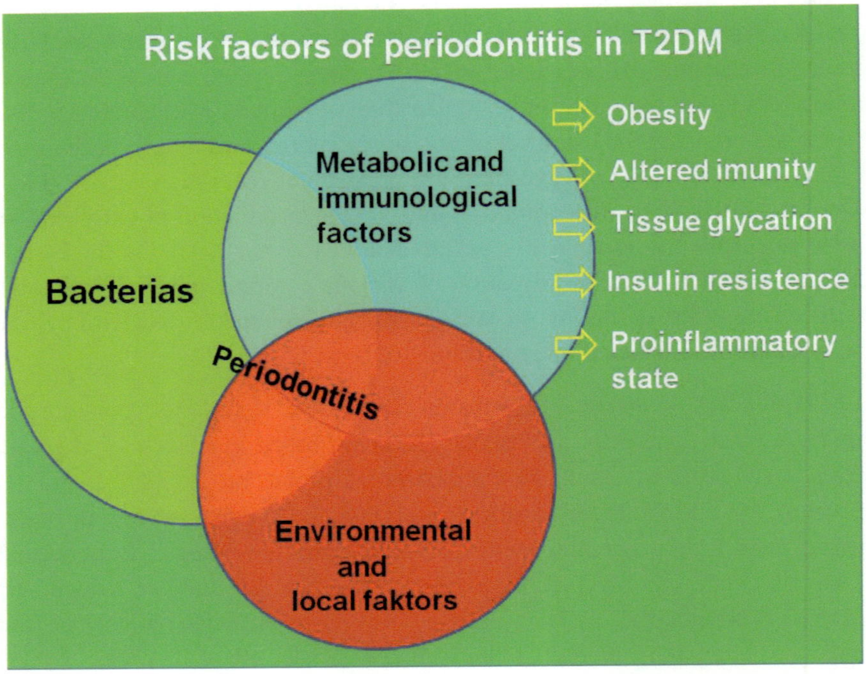

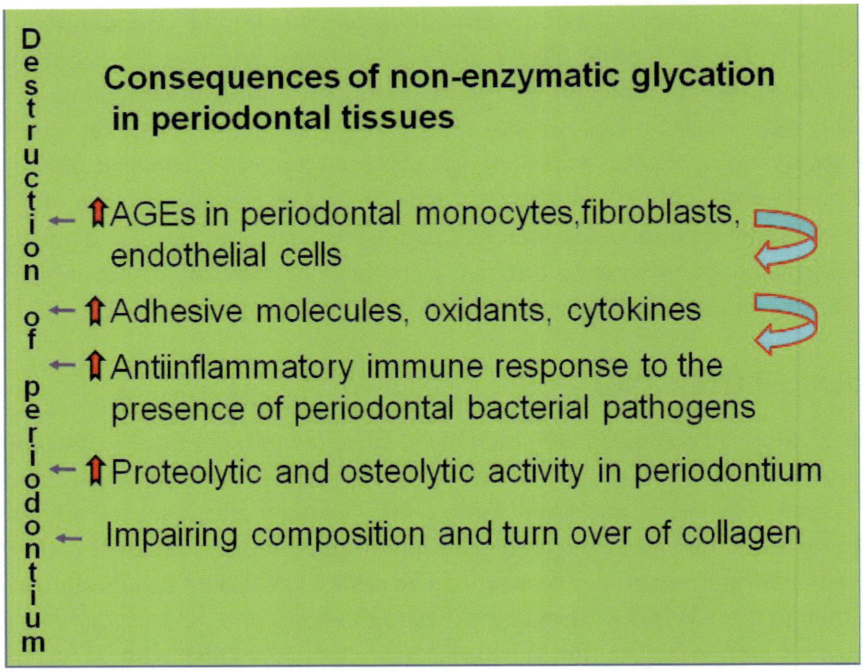

4. Conclusion

From the given knowledge we can summarise several theoretical and practical conclusions which are important for the diabetological and periodontological management of a patient as well as for management of mutual therapeutical associations and procedures:

Patients with diabetes mellitus have twice or three times a larger incidence of periodontitis. This is in relation to significant deterioration of several periodontal parameters such as gingivitis, higher prevalence of periodontal pockets, deeper periodontal pockets, higher BOP score and loss of attachment.

Our present state of knowledge defines DM periodontitis as one of the systemic complications of diabetes though its main etiopathogenic associations in cell-altered immunity, in glycation of periodontal tissues, vascular damage of the periodontium, increased proteolysis and osteolysis of periodontal structures, which result from increased concentrations of pro-inflammatory cytokines, deficient regeneration of collagen structures and quantitative multiplication of periodontal bacterial pathogens.

The level of inflammatory destruction of the periodontium is different in patients with a good level of control of the primary diabetic disease from patients with insufficient control. Changes in periodontal structures can also be detected during the latent stage of diabetes and are reflected in unspecified laboratory and clinical findings.

Nowadays the mutual relationship between these two diseases is considered to run in two directions. Local inflammation in the periodontium significantly influences the systemic disease due to increased susceptibility of the diabetic patient to infection and increased insulin resistance. Deterioration of periodontal parameters and clinical manifestations lead to worsening of the diabetic disease. Without reduction of inflammation in the periodontium we cannot expect any significant improvement of the primary disease.

In collaboration with a diabetologist, we are trying to diagnose gingivitis and periodontitis in the initial stages of diabetes and in detection of the patient's genetic predisposition to diabetic disease.

During treatment of resistant and refractory types of periodontitis, it is necessary to test for diabetic disease, to contact a diabetologist and to try to detect individual pre-diabetic states.

Microbial factors were considerably emphasized in the past. Some studies indicated specific subgingival microflora of some strains, namely P. intermedia and strain capnocytophaga (Khoury et al., 2008). Our current knowledge, described in several studies, indicates that there is no difference in the distribution of individual pathogens in non-diabetic and diabetic patients with periodontitis. However patients with DM are afflicted more often by repeated infectious diseases (Khoury, et al., 2008).

Author details

Michal Straka
Slovak Medical University, Bratislava, Slovakia

Michaela Straka-Trapezanlidis
Private Practice Krizna 44, Bratislava, Slovakia

Acknowledgement

In the chapter, Periodontitis and Diabetes mellitus,, authors deal with mutual relation between both diseases which we percept nowadays as a bidirectional, in the meaning of a mutual reciprocal etiopathogenetic association. They briefly present etiopathogenesis and classification of two main types of diabetes mellitus. The main objective of chapter is to outline and present the mutual etiopathogenetic association. In spite there is not known any distinct causal molecular relation between mentioned diseases in present, exists the certain multifactorial interpretation of mutual pathogenetic coherence in larger epidemiologic, genetic, metabolic, immunologic and therapeutic context. These more specifically defined etiological associations help us as well in diagnostic and therapeutic management in the practice of both diseases, what is emphasized in the conclusion section.

5. References

Al-Zahrani, M.; Bissada, N. & Borawski, A. (2003). Obesity and periodontal disease in young, middle-aged, and older adults. *Journal of Periodontology,* Vo.74, No.5, (May 2OO3), pp. 61O-615, ISSN 0022-3492

Ceriello, A. (2005). Postprandial hyperglycemia and diabetes complications. Is it time to treat ? *Diabetes*, Vol.54, No.1, (January 2005), pp. 1-7, ISSN 0012-1797

Cianciola, J.; Park, B. & Bruck, E. (1982). Prevalence of periodontal disease in insulin-dependent diabetes mellitus (juvenile diabetes). *Journal of American Dental Association,* Vol.104, No.5, (May 1982), pp. 653-660, ISSN 1943-4723

Coenen , K.; Gruen, M. & Chait, A. (2007). Diet-induced increases in adiposity, but not plasma lipids, promote macrophage infiltration into white adipose tissue. *Diabetes,* Vol.56, No. 3, (March 2007), pp. 564-573, ISSN 0012-1797

Collins, S.; Yalda, B. & Arnold, R. (1997). Monotopic TNF-alfa secretions patterns in IDDM patients with periodontal disease *Journal of Clinical Periodontology,* Vol.24, No.1, (January 1997), pp. 8-16, ISSN 0303-6979

Covani, U.; Marconcini, S. & Derchi, G. (2009). Relationship between human periodontitis and type 2 diabetes at a genomic level: A data-mining study. *Journal of Periodontology,* Vol.80, No.8, (August 2009), pp. 1265-1273, ISSN 0022-3492

Covani, U.; Marconcini, S. & Giacomelli, L. (2008). Bioinformatic prediction of leader genes in human periodontitis. *Journal of Periodontology,* Vol.79, No.10, (October 2008), pp. 1974-1983, ISSN 0022-3492

Farkaš, A.; Phillipiová, A. & Ďurovič, E. (2011). Pacient s diagnózou diabetes mellitus zubnej ordinácii. *Stomatológ*, Vol.21, No. 1 (January 2011), pp. 4-10, ISSN 1335-0005

Ferenčík, M. & Hulín, I. (2008). Obezita, tukové tkanivo a zápal. *Medicínsky monitor*, Vol.4, No.1, (January 2008), pp. 1-6, ISSN 1338-2551

Friedlander, AH.; Chaudhuri, G.; Altman l. (2007). A past medical history of gestational diabetes: its medical significance and its dental implications. *Oral Surgery Oral Medicine Oral Pathology Oral Radiology § Endodontics*. Vol.103, No.2, (March 2007), pp. 157-163, ISSN 1528-395X

Galbraith, G.; Steed, R. & Sanders, J. (1998). Tumor necrosis factor alpha production by oral leukocytes: influence of tumor necrosis factor genotype. *Journal of Periodontology*, Vol.69, No.4, (April 1998), pp. 428-433, ISSN 0022-3492

Gislen, G.l; Nilson, KO. & Mattson, L. (1980). Gingival inflammation in diabetic children related to degree of metabolic control. *Acta Odontologica Scandinavica*, Vol.38, No.4, (January 1980), pp. 241-246, ISSN 0001-6357

Kahn, B. & Flier, J. (2000). Obesity and insulin resistance. *Journal of Clinical Investigation*, Vol.106, No.4, (August 2000), pp. 473-481, ISSN 00219738

Kim, J.; Fillmore, J. & Sunshine, M. (2004). PKC-theta knockout mice are protected from fat-induced insulin resistance. *Journal of Clinical Investigation*, Vol.114, No.6, (September 2004), pp. 823-827, ISSN 00219738

King, G. (2008). The role of inflammatory cytokines in diabetes and its complication. *Journal of Periodontology*, Vol. 79, Suppl.8, (August 2008), pp. 1524-1534, ISSN 0022-3492

Khoury, M.; Valdez, R. & Albright, A. (2008). Public health genomic approach to type 2 diabetes. *Diabetes*, Vol.57, No.11, (November 2008), pp. 2911-2914, ISSN 0012-1797

Lambes, F.; Silvestre, F. & Hernandez-Mijares, A. (2008). The effect of periodontal treatment on metabolic control of type 1 diabetes mellitus. *Clinical Oral Investigations*, Vol.12, No.4, (December 2008), pp. 337-343, ISSN 1432-6981

Lyons, T. (1992). Lipoprotein glycation and its metabolic consequences. *Diabetes*, Vol.41, Suppl.2, No.10, (October 1992), pp. 67-70, ISSN 0012-1797

Mandel, R.; Dirienzio, J. & Kent, R. (1992). Microbiology of healthy and diseased periodontal sites in poorly controlled insulin dependent diabetics. *Journal of Periodontology*, Vol.63, No. 4, (April 1992), pp. 274-279, ISSN 0022-3492

McMullen, J.; Van Dyke, T. & Horoszewicz, H. (1981). Neutrophil chemotaxis in individuals with advanced periodontal disease and a genetic predisposition to diabetes mellitus. *Journal of Periodontology*, Vol.52, No.4, (April 1981), pp. 167-171, ISSN 0022-3492

Mealey, B. & Oates, T. (2006). Diabetas mellitus and periodontal diseases. AAP-Commisssioned review. *Journal of Periodontology*, Vol.77, No.8, (August 2006), pp. 1289-1303, ISSN 0022-3492

Mehta, N.; McGillicuddy, F. & Anderson, P. (2010). Experimental endotoxemia induces adipose inflammation and insulin resistance in humans. *Diabetes*. Vol.59, No.1, (January 2010), pp. 172-181, ISSN 0012-1797

Nelson, RG.; Schlossman, M. & Budding, L. (1990). Periodontal disease and NIDDM in Pima indians. *Diabetes Care*, Vol.13, No.8, (August 1990), pp. 836-840, ISSN 0149-5992

Nishimura, F.; Iwamoto, Y. & Mineshiba, J. (2003). Periodontal disease and diabetes mellitus: The role of tumor necrosis factor-alfa in a 2-way relationship. *Journal of Periodontology*, Vol.74, No.1, (January 2003), pp. 97-102, ISSN 0022-3492

Novak, KF.; Taylor, GW.; Dawson, DR.; Ferguson II, JE.; Novak, MJ. (2006). Periodontitis and Gestational Diabetes Mellitus: Exploring the link in NHANES III. *Journal of Public Health Dentistry*, Vol. 66, No.3, (March 2006), pp. 163-168, ISSN 0022-4006

Rybka, J. (1990). *Pokroky v diabetologii I.*, pp. 21-39, ISBN 8020100407, Prague, Czech Republic

Salvi ,GE.; Collins, JG. & Yalda, B. (1997). Monocytic TNF-alfa secretion patterns in IDDM patients with periodontal disease. *Journal of Clinical Periodontology*, Vol.24, No.1 (January 1997), pp. 8-18, ISSN 0303-6979

Shoelson, S.; Jongsoon, L. & Goldifine, A. (2006). Inflammation and insulin resistance. *Journal of Clinical Investigation*, Vol.116, No.7, (July 2006), pp. 1793-1801, ISSN 00219738

Shulman, G. (2000). Cellular mechanisms of insulin resistance. *Journal of Clinical Investigation*, Vol.106, No. 2, (July 2000), pp. 171-179, ISSN 00219738

Straka, M. (2001). Parodontitis a diabetes mellitus. *Progresdent*, Vol.6, (Jun 2001), pp. 10-12, ISSN 1211-3859

Straka, M. (2011). Oral manifestations of diabetes mellitus and influences of periodontolological treatment on diabetes mellitus. *Bratislava Medical Journal*, Vol. 7, No. 112, (July 2011), pp. 416-420, ISSN 0006-9248

Straka, M; Trapezanlidis, M; Kotráň, M. (2011). Periodontitis and preterm low birth weight: Is there any associations? *Journal of Reproductive system and sexual disorders*. Special Issue: Operative Gynecology & High Risk Pregnancy S2:002, ISSN: 2161-038X

Tervonen, T.; Lamminsalo, S. & Hiltunen, L. (2009). Resolution of periodontal inflammation does not guarentee improved glycemic control in type 1 diabetic subjects. *Journal of Clinical Periodontology*, Vol.36, No.1, (January 2009), pp. 51-57, ISSN 0303-6979

Tsai, C.; Hayes, C. & Taylor, GV.(2002). Glycemic control of type 2 diabetes and severe periodontal disease in the US adult population. *Community of Dental and Oral Epidemiology*, Vol.3O, No.3, (June 2002), pp. 182-192, ISSN 0301-5661

Watanabe, K.; Petro, B. & Shlimon, A. (2008). Effects of periodontitis on insulin resistance and the onset of type 2 diabetes mellitus in Zucker diabetic fatty rats. *Journal of Periodontology*, Vol.79, No.7, (July 2008), pp. 1208-1216, ISSN 0022-3492

Xiong, X.; Buekens, P.; Vatardis, S.; Pridjian, G. (2006). Periodontal disease and gestational diabetes mellitus. *American Journal of Obstetrics § Gynecology*, Vol. 195, No.4 (October 2006), pp.1086-1089, ISSN 0002-9378

Zambon, J.; Reynolds, H. & Fisher, J. (1988). Microbiological and immunological studies of adult periodontitis in patients with noninsulin-dependent diabetes mellitus. *Journal of Periodontology*, Vol.59, No.1, (January 1988), pp. 23-31, ISSN 0022-3492